I0440369

Introduction to the book

Are you a fan of oats? Do you want to know what benefits oats offer to your body? So go ahead and read this valuable book to learn about the full benefits of oats.

Let us learn in the following about the benefits of oats and many important information about it:

The benefits of oats
The health and nutritional benefits of oats lie in the fact that it contains complete dietary fiber and many essential and important vitamins and minerals. One cup of oats contains approximately 26 micrograms of folic acid, and more than 10 grams of protein.

The most prominent benefits of oats are as follows:
1. Promote cardiovascular health
One of the most important benefits of oats is that it enhances the health of the heart and arteries, due to the fact that oats contain:

1

Soluble dietary fiber

Where these fibers prevent the absorption of low-density lipoprotein, which is known as bad cholesterol (LDL), and this promotes cardiovascular health and reduces the risk of high blood pressure.

Antioxidant Avenanthramides

Afanthramide antioxidant prevents the production of harmful molecules, which stick to the walls of the arteries and are deposited on them and may be the cause of their narrowing and thus lead to hardening and thrombosis of the arteries, and with the presence of this antioxidant they are fought and thus prevent atherosclerosis.

2. Preventing weight gain

Oatmeal is one of the good whole grains in preventing weight gain, due to its composition, as it contain

Low in calories: one portion of it gives approximately 80 calories.

A high percentage of dietary fiber: which works to increase the feeling of satiety for a longer period, which reduces food intake and thus reduces the percentage of calories entering the body.

A good percentage of protein: Protein also supports the matter of increasing the feeling of satiety for a long time, and thus reducing the amount of food eaten later.

3. Diabetes prevention

One of the benefits of oats is to maintain and control blood sugar levels, for several reasons, namely:

It contains a large amount of complex carbohydrates and beneficial dietary fibers, as this helps slow the absorption of sugar in the intestine and regulate its level in the blood, and thus plays an important role in preventing type 2 diabetes.

It contains magnesium, which helps regulate insulin and glucose levels in the body

4. Strengthening immunity

Oatmeal can strengthen the immune system, as it contains a type of fiber known as beta gluten that helps boost immunity and fight infection.

5. Contributing to the prevention of cancer

It was previously mentioned that oats contain an antioxidant called afanthramide, and this antioxidant works to fight free radicals that may cause some infections and cancers.

Oatmeal has also been linked to preventing the development of breast cancer and fighting it, as it is one of the whole grains that contain the necessary and important fibers to combat carcinogens, in addition to containing some substances that reduce the level of estrogen in the body.

Ways to eat oats

To obtain the benefits of oats, it can be eaten in one of the following ways:

Ready-made chips. It is preferable to eat this type for breakfast.

Whole grains added to some foods such as milk and some soups.

Cereals mixed with different fruits, such as apples, cranberries, and strawberries.

Flour in some baked goods and sweets.

Harmful effects of oats

Despite the benefits of oats, eating large amounts of it may lead to harm for some, and these damages are as follows:

Allergy to oats: Many people suffer from allergies immediately after eating oats, which appears in the form of a runny nose, rash, and high body temperature.

Digestive disorders: It often occurs to people who suffer from digestive problems, such as: patients with irritable bowel syndrome, so it is preferable to stay away from these groups.

Choking: This happens if taken in the form of whole grains, so it is recommended to chew it well before swallowing, or take it in the form of flour

Benefits of oatsget to know them

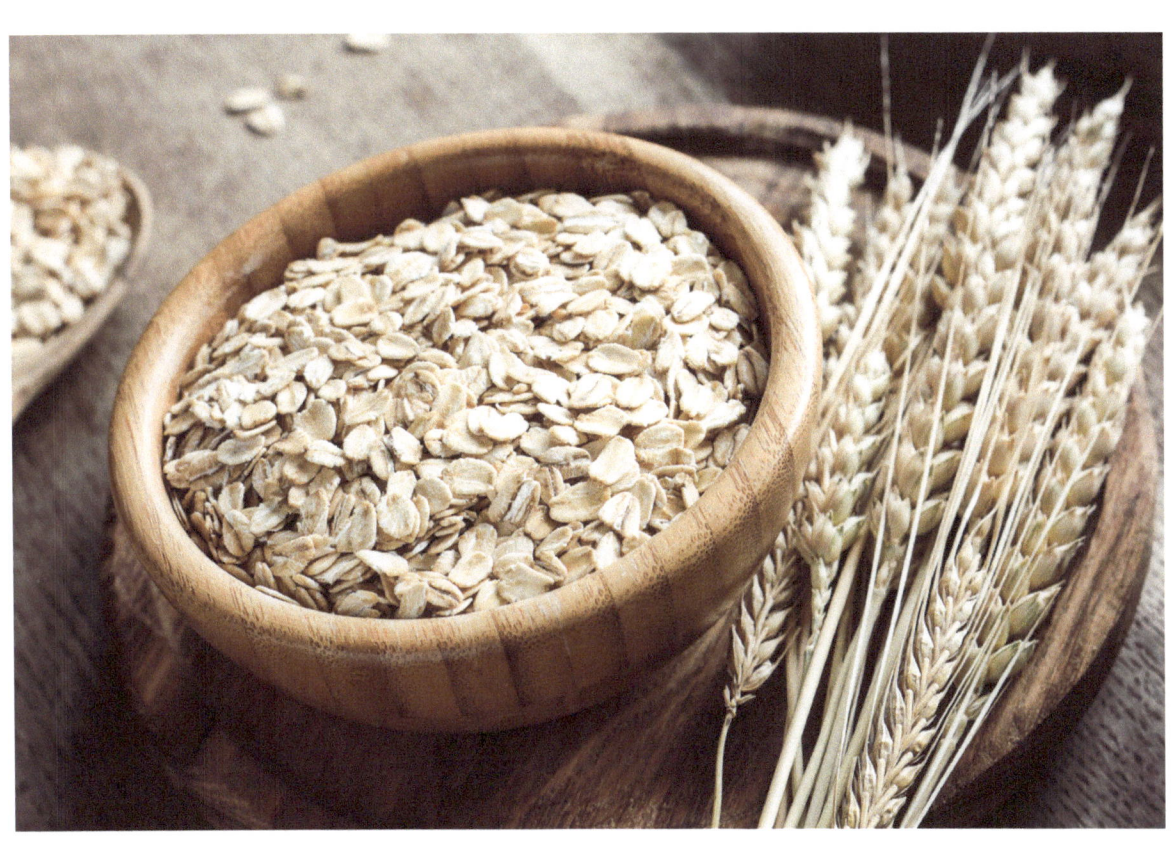

Are you a fan of oats? Do you want to know what benefits oats offer to your body? So read the article to learn about the full benefits of oats.

Let us know what follows about the benefits of oats and many important information about it

The benefits of oats

The health and nutritional benefits of oats lie in the fact that it contains complete dietary fiber and many essential and important vitamins and minerals . One cup of oats contains approximately 26 micrograms of folic acid, and more than 10 grams of protein.

The most important benefits of oats are as follows:

1. Promote cardiovascular health

One of the most important benefits of oats is that it enhances the health of the heart and arteries, due to the fact that oats contain:

Soluble dietary fibre

Where these fibers prevent the absorption of low-density lipoprotein, which is known as bad cholesterol (LDL), and this promotes cardiovascular health and reduces the risk of high blood pressure.

Antioxidant Avenanthramides

Afanthramide antioxidant prevents the production of harmful molecules, which stick to the walls of the arteries and are deposited on them and may be the cause of their narrowing and thus lead to hardening and thrombosis of the arteries, and with the presence of this antioxidant they are fought and thus prevent atherosclerosis.

2. Prevention of weight gain

Oatmeal is one of the good whole grains in preventing weight gain, due to its composition, as it contains:

Low in calories: one portion of it gives approximately 80 calories.

A high percentage of dietary fiber: which works to increase the feeling of satiety for a longer period, which reduces food intake and thus reduces the percentage of calories entering the body.

A good percentage of protein: Protein also supports the matter of increasing the feeling of satiety for a long time, and thus reducing the amount of food eaten later.

3. Diabetes prevention

One of the benefits of oats is to maintain and control blood sugar levels, for several reasons, namely:

It contains a large amount of complex carbohydrates and beneficial dietary fibers , as this helps slow the absorption of sugar in the intestine and regulate its level in the blood, and thus plays an important role in preventing type 2 diabetes.

It contains magnesium, which helps regulate insulin and glucose levels in the body.

4. Strengthening immunity

Oatmeal can strengthen the immune system , as it contains a type of fiber known as beta gluten, which helps boost immunity and fight infection.

5. Contribute to the prevention of cancer

It was previously mentioned that oats contain an antioxidant called afanthramide, and this antioxidant works to fight free radicals that may cause some infections and cancers.

Oatmeal has also been linked to preventing the development of breast cancer and fighting it, as it is one of the whole grains that contain the necessary and important fibers to combat carcinogens, in addition to containing some substances that reduce the level of estrogen in the body.

Ways to eat oats
To obtain the benefits of oats, it can be eaten in one of the following ways:

Ready-made chips, and it is preferable to eat this type for breakfast.
Whole grains are added to some foods, such as milk and some soups.
Cereal mixed with different fruits, such as: apples, cranberries , and strawberries.
Flour in some baked goods and desserts.

Oat damage

Despite the benefits of oats, eating large amounts of it may lead to harm for some, and these damages are as follows:

Allergy to oats: Many people suffer from allergies immediately after eating oats, which appears in the form of a runny nose, rash , and high body temperature.

Digestive disorders: It often occurs to people who suffer from digestive problems , such as: patients with irritable bowel syndrome, so it is preferable to stay away from these groups.

Choking: This happens if taken in the form of whole grains, so it is recommended to chew it well before swallowing, or take it in the form of flour.

What happens to your body when you eat oats daily?

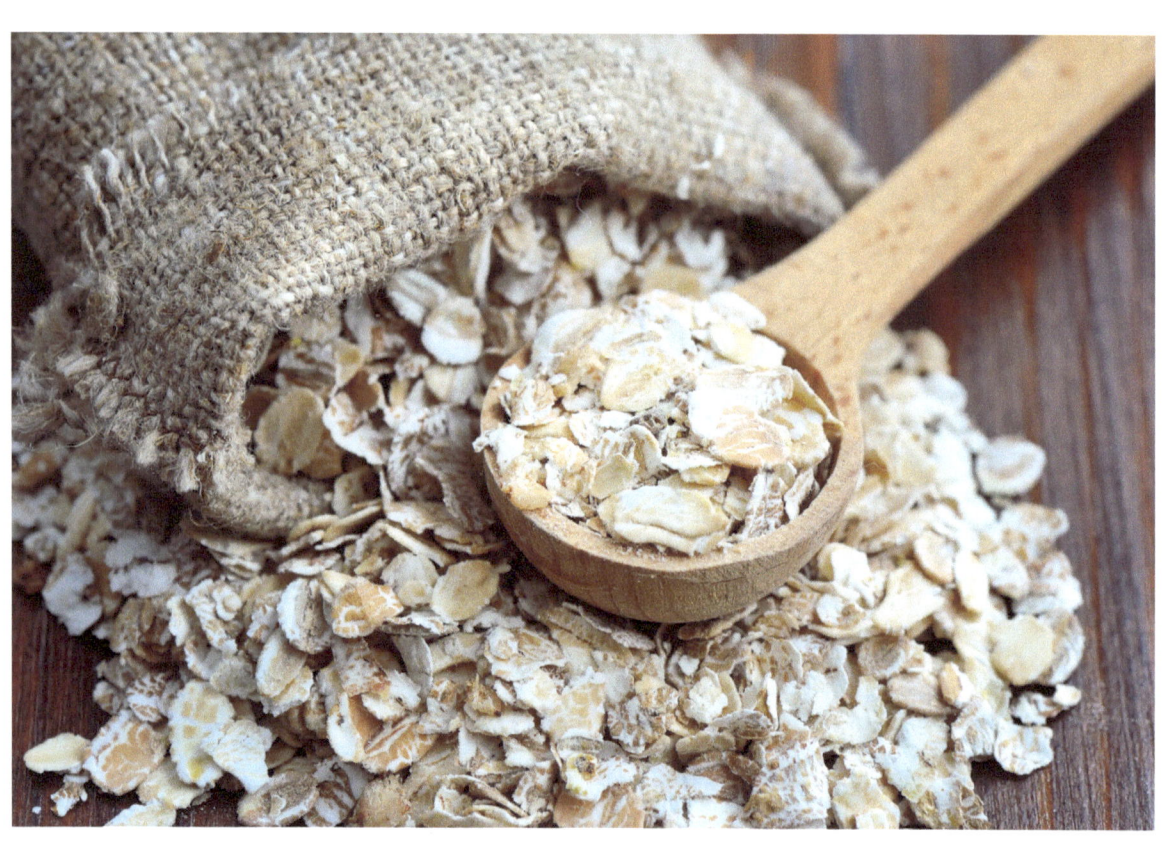

Oatmeal is one of the whole grains that has recently become famous for its many benefits to the body. Have you ever thought about what happens to your body when you eat oats daily?

Oatmeal is one of the whole grains that can be an ideal, healthy, quick-to-prepare breakfast with great nutritional value if consumed regularly. Let us introduce you to the benefits of eating oatmeal daily in the following.

Benefits of eating oats daily
Among the benefits of oats as a daily meal:

source of energy

Eating a meal of oatmeal for breakfast provides a large amount of energy that will continue with you during the day, and will help you to accomplish your daily activities without getting tired. The reason for this is:

1-High content of dietary fiber, which is a complex carbohydrate that helps regulate blood sugar levels, increase satiety and give you more energy for a long time.

2-Oatmeal is high in B vitamins, which contribute to enhancing energy production in the body.

Reducing the risk of obesity

One of the benefits of oats as a daily meal is to reduce the risk of obesity. This is due to its high content of dietary fiber , which helps to fill the stomach and increase the sense of satiety.

Compared to breakfast cereal made with cornflakes, oatmeal is slower digested and therefore:

1-Reduces the feeling of hunger.
2-Reduce the amount of meals eaten later.
3-It reduces calories and prevents weight gain and obesity.
Diabetes prevention
Eating oats daily helps prevent type 2 diabetes, as it has a low glycemic index (an indicator of high blood sugar).

When the glycemic index of food is low, this means that the gastric emptying process will be slower, and thus this will affect blood sugar levels and will improve insulin sensitivity.
This was confirmed by the results of a study published in the American Journal of Clinical Nutrition, that eating foods with a lower glycemic index is associated with less insulin resistance and a lower risk of type 2 diabetes.

Promote heart health
One of the benefits of oats as a daily meal is promoting heart health.

Many studies have linked the consumption of oats with the promotion of heart health, due to its high content of dietary fiber, in addition to being a rich source of vitamins and minerals important for regulating the work of the heart.

And it was found in a study published in the American Journal of Clinical Nutrition that eating whole grain meals reduces the risk of coronary heart disease.

It has also been shown that beta-glucan, one of the most important soluble fibers present in oats, has a positive effect on reducing cholesterol.

Promote skin health

Oatmeal is an ideal food to promote skin and skin health and care for it, and it is considered soothing and relieving irritations and itching, as oatmeal helps to adjust the pH of the skin.

The American Academy of Dermatology recommends using oatmeal to treat various skin conditions, including eczema.

Great nutritional value

Eating oats daily is very beneficial as oats are a great source of a large number of different nutrients required for a healthy body, such as:

1-Complex carbohydrates , vegetable proteins and little fat.

2-Many important minerals and vitamins such as iron, copper, phosphorous , calcium and zinc.

Reducing the risk of asthma in children

Studies have shown that feeding infants younger than 6 months old with oats reduced their risk of childhood asthma.

Reducing constipation

Eating oats daily is beneficial for constipation, as it was found that oat bran reduced constipation in the elderly, and also reduced their need for laxatives.

Oats with milkdon't miss out on their benefits

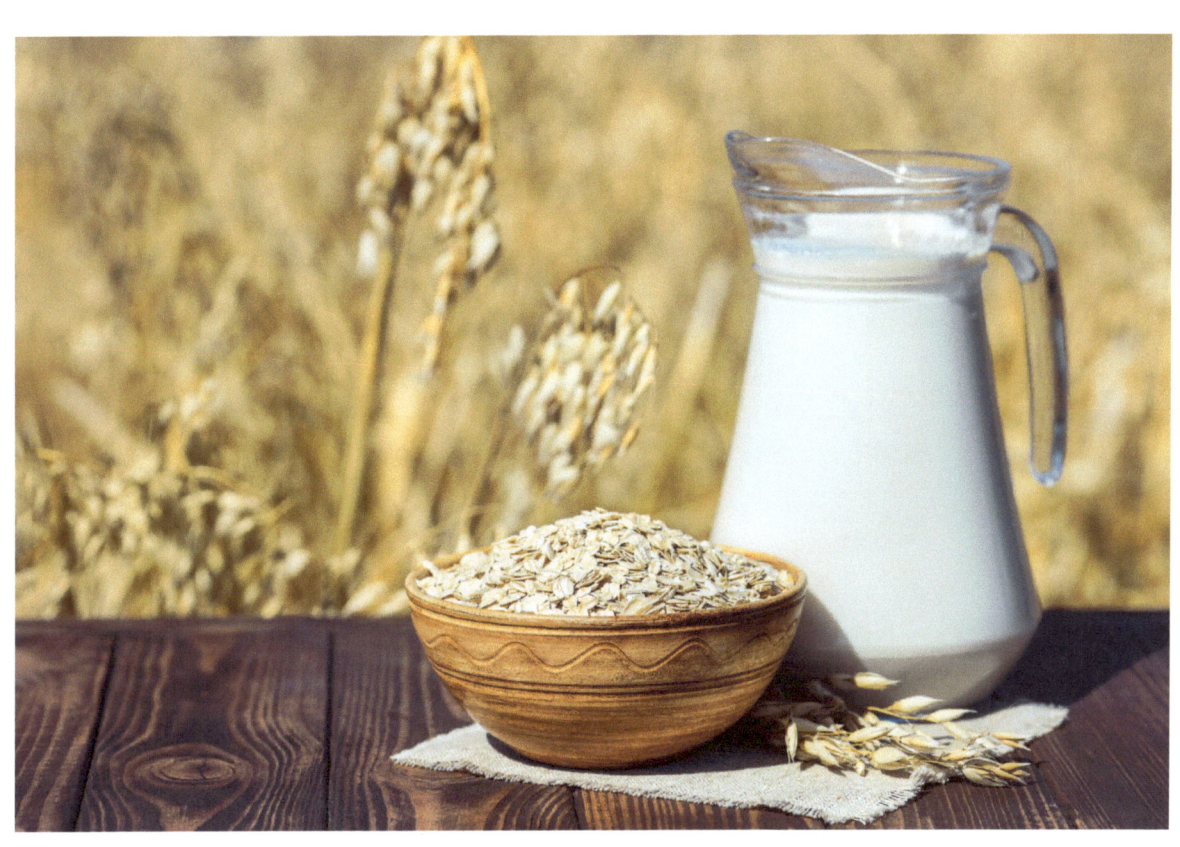

Oatmeal with milk is everyone's favorite breakfast, but what are its benefits? How can it be prepared?

Oatmeal with milk is one of the healthy foods that can be eaten at breakfast. It provides the body with energy and satiety for long periods because it is a whole grain. In the following article, we will get to know oats with milk better.

Benefits of oats with milk

There are many benefits of oats with milk besides the delicious taste, and among these benefits we mention:

1. It improves cholesterol levels

Oats contain a type of fiber called beta-glucan that improves cholesterol levels, by lowering the bad LDL cholesterol level.

2. Regulates blood sugar levels

One of the benefits of oats is regulating blood sugar levels; It improves the body's reaction to insulin due to its beta-glucan content, and this benefit can be obtained by eating oatmeal with milk without adding sugar.

3. Rich in antioxidants

Eating oats with milk provides many beneficial antioxidants for the body, such as polyphenols rich in avenanthramides, which offer many benefits, including:

Increase nitric acid production, which regulates blood pressure.

Promote blood flow in the body.

Reducing inflammation and itching.

4. Helps regulate weight

One of the benefits of oatmeal with milk is weight regulation. As oats provide the body with soluble fibers that increase the feeling of fullness in individuals and reduce the desire to eat other foods for a period of not less than 4 hours.

5. Rich in salts and vitamins

Oats with milk are an important source of many minerals such as magnesium, iron, zinc, folic acid and phosphorus.

It is also a rich source of B vitamins essential for brain health, vitamin B1, which is needed for converting glucose into energy, vitamin B5, which is needed for the production of acetylcholine, which is necessary for memory and learning, and vitamin B6, which is necessary for converting tryptophan into serotonin .

6. It prevents constipation

One of the benefits of oats is to regulate bowel movement naturally, as it contains soluble fiber that may prevent constipation.

How to prepare oats with milk

Oatmeal is prepared with milk instead of water to get the maximum benefit from the feeling of satiety resulting from the proteins found in milk. Oatmeal can be prepared with milk by following the following steps:

1-Put a cup and a half of milk with a small pinch of salt in a saucepan over the fire.

2-Add half a cup of oats, and if you want the texture of the oats with milk to be creamy, you should add the oats after boiling the milk, but if you want the oats to maintain their consistency, you should add the oats to the cold milk.

3-Stir the mixture, then reduce the heat when the milk begins to boil, and stir for about 5 minutes, or until the oats absorb the milk.

4-Put the oats with milk in a plate, and add any other ingredients you want to add.

Tips for preparing oatmeal with milk

There are several tips that can be followed to get the greatest possible benefit from oatmeal with milk, and among these tips we mention:

Make sure to get gluten-free oats in the event of a gluten-free diet , knowing that the oats themselves are gluten-free, but gluten may be added during the manufacturing or packaging process.

Use unsweetened milk, or you can use almond milk or coconut milk if you are lactose intolerant .

The necessity of continuous stirring of the mixture until the oats excrete the starch present in it in the event that a thick consistency is desired.

Another source of protein can be added to your oats with milk, such as nuts or seeds.

You can add some dried fruits or spices such as cinnamon or ginger, which add a delicious taste to oatmeal with milk and increase its nutritional value.

Does oatmeal gain weight? Here's the answer

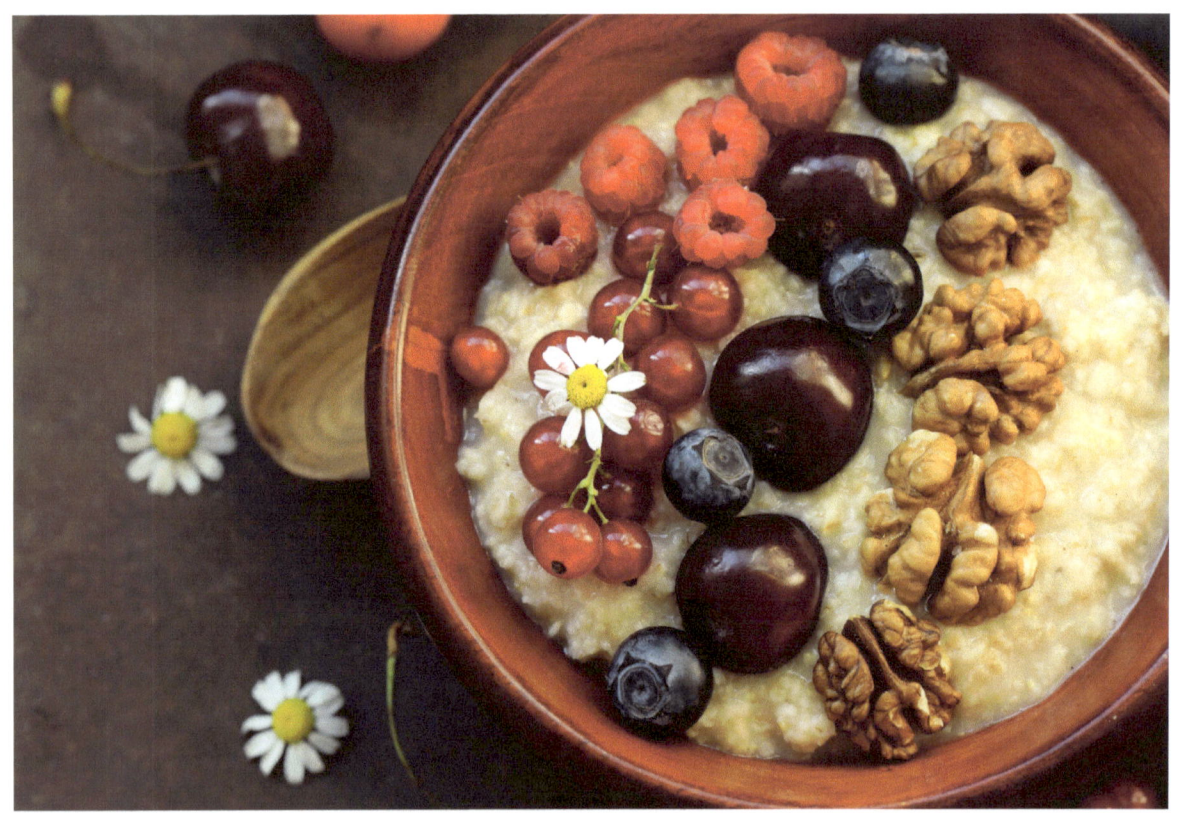

Oatmeal is used as one of the main healthy diets, but does oatmeal make you gain weight?

Oats contribute to reducing the risk of heart disease and help control blood pressure, but what does oats have to do with weight gain? Does oatmeal increase weight? The answers and more are as follows:

Does oatmeal gain weight?
Oatmeal is one of the types of cereals rich in dietary fiber , which contains a set of properties that make it beneficial for the health of the body.

Oats play an important role in weight loss diets, but do oats make you gain weight? Yes, oats are characterized as a double-edged sword, as they can increase weight and have a role in losing it, and that depends on how and how much oats are eaten.

Here are some of the ways oats make you gain weight:

1. Eat plenty of oats

The increase in the consumption of any type of food makes the food unhealthy for the body, as well as oats. Increasing the consumption of oats for the normal amount per meal may lead to weight gain.

Therefore, it is important to determine the amount of an individual's daily meal of oats to prevent weight gain from it if he does not want the opposite, as there are people trying to gain weight.

2. Combine oats with other foods

Does oatmeal gain weight? Yes, if some foods that lead to weight gain are added to it, as chocolate is added to oats in breakfast meals .

These additives that lead to weight gain can be replaced with many fresh fruits, such as: berries, pomegranates, and strawberries .

Oatmeal, milk and banana recipe

It is a very effective recipe for weight gain, and to prepare it, the following steps are followed:

1-Each of the following ingredients is prepared:

A glass of liquid milk.

A quarter cup of oats.

Banana cut into rings.

Two tablespoons of peanut butter .

One tablespoon of honey.

Nuts for decoration.

2-The milk is placed on a medium heat until it reaches a boil.

3-Add the oats to the milk for about 5-7 minutes.

4-Oatmeal is poured into a serving dish, and banana rings, peanut butter, honey, and nuts are distributed on it.

5-The dish is served immediately.

So, as mentioned earlier, the answer to the question, do oats make you gain weight? Yes, depending on how you use it and how you set it up.

Oatmeal dietyour way to lose weight

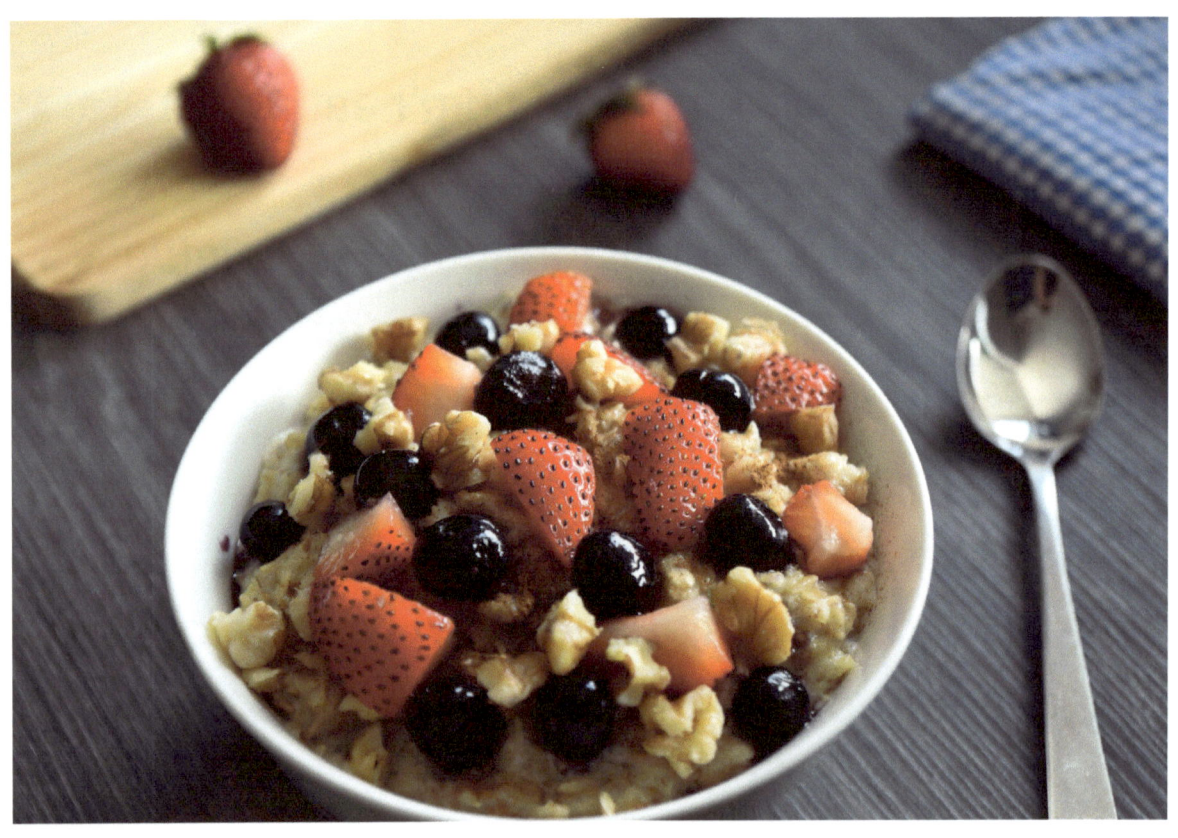

Due to the nutritional importance of oats, it can be followed as a diet to reduce weight. What is the oatmeal diet? How can it be followed?

We often hear many recipes and ways to lose weight, and one of them is the use of oatmeal, so what is the oatmeal diet ? Can it help you lose weight?

What is the oat diet?

If you want to follow the oatmeal diet to reduce your weight, you can follow the following diet:

1. Breakfast

You can have a morning snack that contains fresh fruits, or some raw vegetables, and add oats to it, and you can add a small amount of oats to skim milk and low-fat yogurt, and cinnamon is a great addition to the flavor.

It should be noted that the oatmeal should be whole and not instant; Because instant oats often contain added sugar.

2. Lunch

The recommended serving size is ½ cup of oatmeal at lunch with your main meals.

3. Dinner

This meal usually includes grilled chicken, fish , a light lean steak, or even a turkey burger, and the oats are added along with the vegetables as they cook with the meal.

Preparing oats for the diet

The most common way to use oats is to eat it with milk and add some nuts and fruits to enhance its taste. Here are simple ways to prepare oats for the diet:

Prepare oatmeal with half a cup of water or low-fat milk.

Mix the oats with boiling water until the oats become soft, and then add some nuts and fruits to it.

Adding oats to baked goods.

How does the oatmeal diet help lose weight?

Oatmeal is a healthy and beneficial breakfast option for reducing body weight, as it works on the following:

1. Reducing the level of sugar in the blood

People with diabetes suffer from irregular blood sugar levels as a result of decreased sensitivity of cells to insulin.

One of the benefits of oatmeal is to increase cell response to insulin, thus helping to control blood sugar levels.

2. Reducing cholesterol levels and harmful fats in the blood
Studies have shown the significant role of beta-glucan fiber found in oats in lowering blood cholesterol and preventing body fat from oxidation.

3. Oats contain important nutrients
Oats are an important part of a healthy diet, as half a cup of oats cooked in water contains very few calories, in addition to the following nutritional values:

fiber2 gr	
proteins3 gr	
sugars0 gr	
Fats1.5 gr	
calcium2% of the daily recommended amount	
Iron6% of the daily recommended amount	

4. Feeling full for long periods

Oatmeal helps control the amount of food intake by giving a longer feeling of satiety.

The dangers of the oat diet

Oats offer a number of benefits to your health, but there are some risks that you should pay attention to, especially when following an oat diet, including:

The oatmeal diet can cause malnutrition for you, as it is a very low-calorie diet, and it does not provide the nutrients that a person needs on a daily basis.
The oatmeal diet can make you feel hungry, dizzy, and tired.
It can cause difficulty in maintaining weight loss.
It can exacerbate some diseases and cause other health problems, such as: kidney stones and gout.
It can increase the risk of chronic health problems, such as: heart disease, high blood pressure, osteoporosis, and cancers.
But adding lean protein, fruits, vegetables, whole grains, and healthy fats to your oatmeal diet can help reduce these risks.

Benefits of oats for athletes

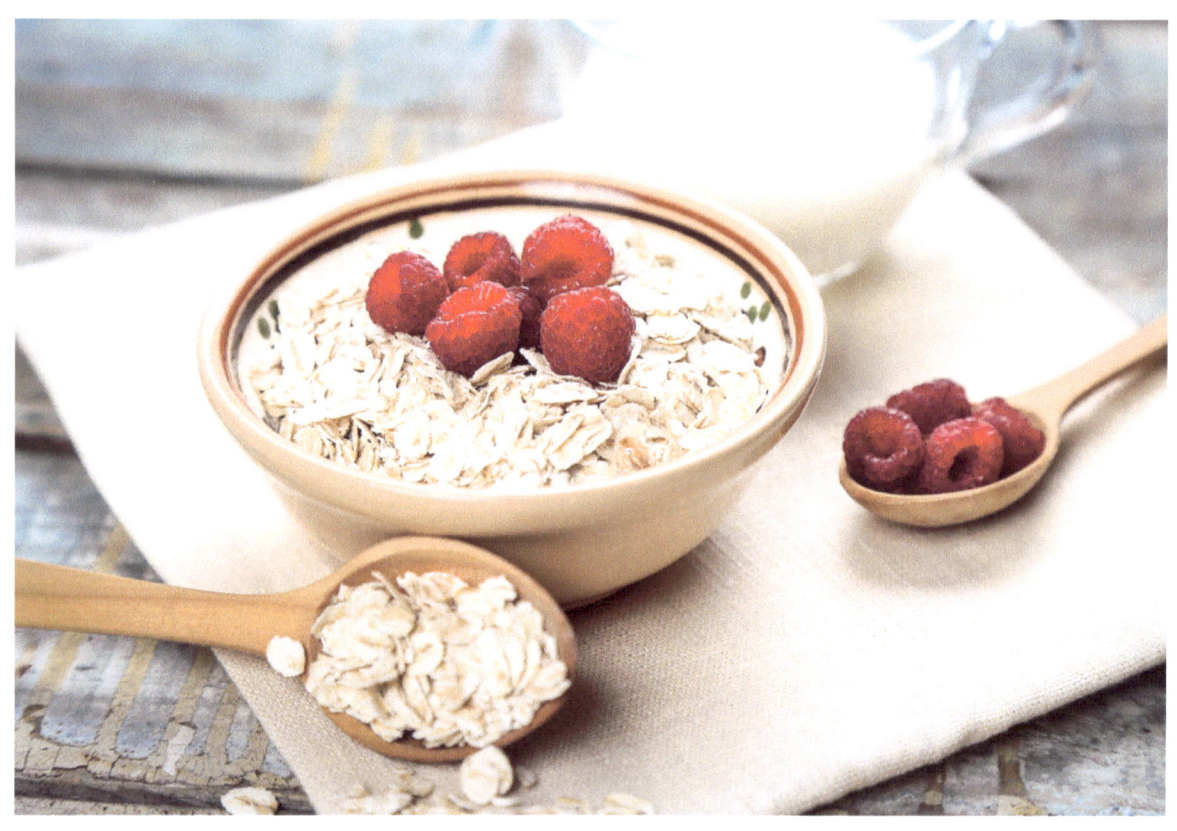

Oatmeal is one of the healthy meals that can be eaten early in the morning, so what are the most important benefits of oatmeal for athletes?

Oats contain proteins and many important nutrients, so what are the most important benefits of oats for athletes?

Benefits of oats for athletes
Here are the most important benefits of oats for athletes:

1. A good source of proteins
Oatmeal is one of the sources rich in protein that is important for building muscle for people who exercise regularly, as one cup of oatmeal contains 166 calories, 4 grams of fiber, and 6 grams of protein.

Oats contain more protein than any other grain, so oats are a good source of protein and are useful for building muscle.

2. Rich in important nutrients

Oats contain iron and B vitamins that are important for the body, in addition to beneficial fiber.

3. Provide athletes with energy

Oats contain iron, which is important for transporting oxygen throughout the body and to various organs in order to produce energy . You can obtain 46% of the iron required daily by eating one serving of oats.

Oats also contain the carbohydrates needed to produce energy in athletes, which makes oats a good choice to eat early in the morning or before exercising.

4. Providing a person with satiety for a long time

Oats contain a type of fiber called beta-glucan, which in turn is responsible for the viscosity and thickness of oats when water is added to them, in addition to giving athletes a feeling of fullness for a long time.

5. Increase the burn rate

When eating complex carbohydrates, such as those found in oats, the body increases the burning rate significantly, which also means its ability to burn fat in athletic people.

6. Helps sleep

Although most people eat oatmeal for breakfast, eating it for dinner greatly helps with sleep, as sleeping for sufficient hours is one of the main factors that helps athletic people do various exercises.

Oats contain melatonin and complex carbohydrates that help deliver a greater amount of tryptophan to the brain, which in turn helps with sleep.
Oats also contain B vitamins, which help secrete a greater amount of serotonin, thus stimulating sleep.

How to prepare oatmeal for athletes

Cooking whole oats requires a little time, unlike rolled or cracked oats, which require less preparation time.

Sports people can prepare oatmeal the way they prefer and add cow's milk , plant milk, or water to it.

Preparing oatmeal often takes 10–60 minutes, depending on the type of oatmeal. The following are the most important steps to do so:

1-Boil 1.5 cups of your favorite milk or water.
2-Add 1/2 cup of oats to the pot containing milk or boiling water.
3-Reduce heat to medium.
4-Leave the oats on the stove for 10–20 minutes for split or ground oats, or 50–60 minutes for whole oats.
5-Add any of your favorite ingredients to oatmeal, such as: cinnamon or honey.
6-Instant oats can be used, but these are often refined and contain sugars and preservatives.\

Side effects of oats

Oats are considered safe when taken orally in reasonable amounts, but eating them in large quantities leads to symptoms related to the digestive system, such as: gas and bloating.

It is recommended to eat oats in a small amount when eating it for the first time, and then gradually increase the amount until it reaches the required amount, as the body requires some time to get used to digesting oats due to the amount of fiber present in it.

Benefits of oats for muscles

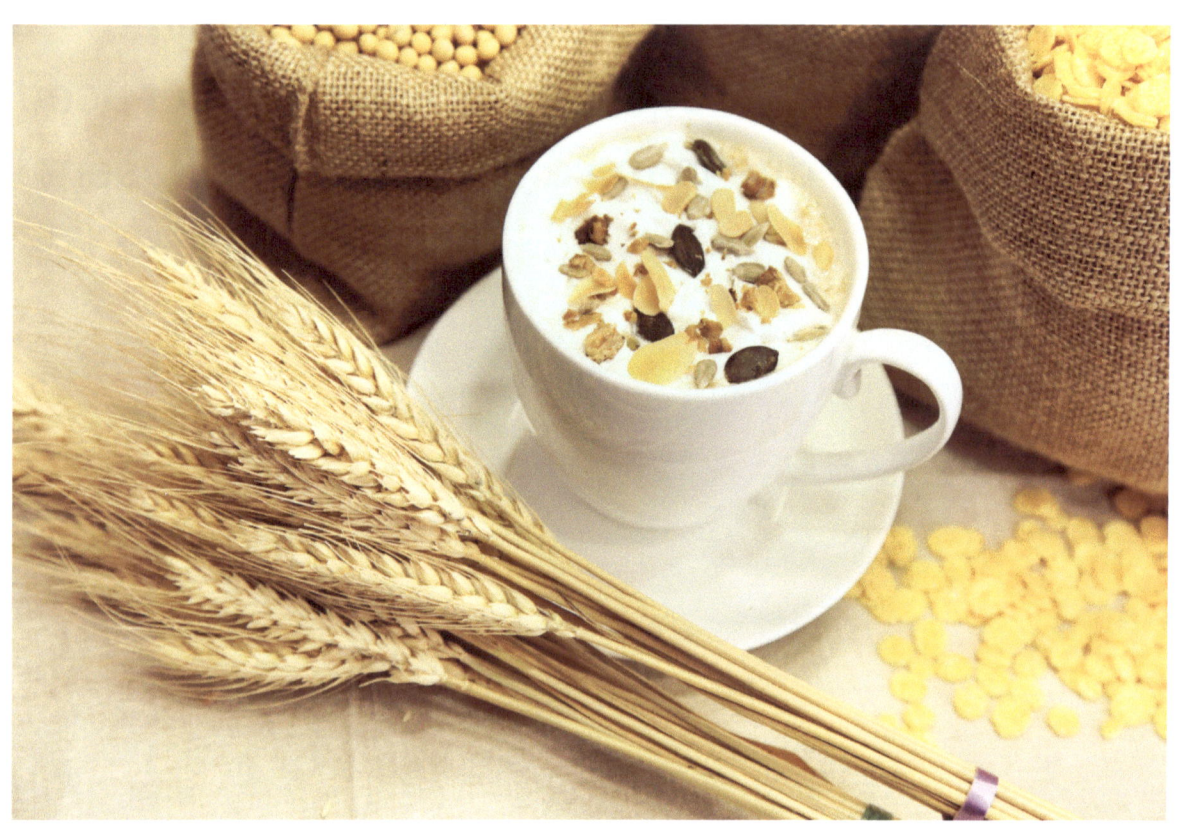

Most athletes prefer to eat oatmeal or add it to different meals, especially in the early morning. What are the most important benefits of oatmeal for muscles?

Oatmeal is one of the healthy ingredients rich in minerals and proteins, so what are the most important benefits of oatmeal for muscles?

Benefits of oatmeal for muscles

Oatmeal has many benefits for human health because it contains vitamins, minerals and beneficial nutrients. Here are the most important benefits of oatmeal for muscles:

1. A source of complex carbohydrates

Athletes are often advised to choose sources of complex carbohydrates as a source of energy instead of sources of quickly absorbed carbohydrates, as the complex carbohydrates found in oats give people energy to build muscles when they want to do muscle-building exercises, as carbohydrates help to enlarge muscles in the human body, because proteins It alone is not sufficient to do this.

It should be noted that the complex carbohydrates found in oats do not significantly raise insulin levels, which means that they provide satiety for a person for a long period of time.

2. Promote muscle building

One cup of oats contains 41.6 milligrams of magnesium, which is one of the important elements that helps build muscles in the human body.

3. Relieve muscle tension

Because oats contain magnesium, it plays an important role in maintaining muscle comfort after exercise, and thus it protects people from muscle strain. [Reference]

4. Maintaining muscle health

Oats are one of the types of foods rich in proteins, as 40 grams of oats contain about 7 grams of protein. Adding oats to the daily diet helps provide the human body with the proteins necessary to maintain muscle health and repair damaged muscle cells. [Reference]

Oats are also one of the types of foods rich in iron, as iron helps produce red blood cells that transport oxygen to all muscles and organs of the body and rid them of waste, thus maintaining their health.

Ways to eat oats

One of the best things about oats is that it can be eaten with salty or sweet dishes, and it can also be eaten daily and added to different meals, as follows:

1-Most people prefer to eat oatmeal for breakfast, but it can also be eaten before or after a workout.

2-Many oatmeal recipes can be prepared by adding all kinds of milk, such as: almond milk or coconut milk. You can also add milk and different types of fruits, such as: bananas, strawberries, berries, nuts or cheese at times.

3-Some prepare savory meals or soups that also contain oats, with the addition of spinach, onions, or any type of vegetable. [Reference]

Side effects of oats

After learning about the benefits of oatmeal for muscles, it is worth noting its harms and precautions for its use.

Oral oatmeal is considered safe, especially when eaten in reasonable quantities and within the normal meal rate, but eating oats in huge and large quantities leads to some side effects related to the digestive system, such as: gas and bloating, and this is due to the fact that oats contain a large amount of fiber. .

Therefore, it is recommended to eat oats in very small quantities at first and then gradually increase the amount to the required amount in order to avoid most of the side effects associated with oats.

Oat bread: many benefits for your health

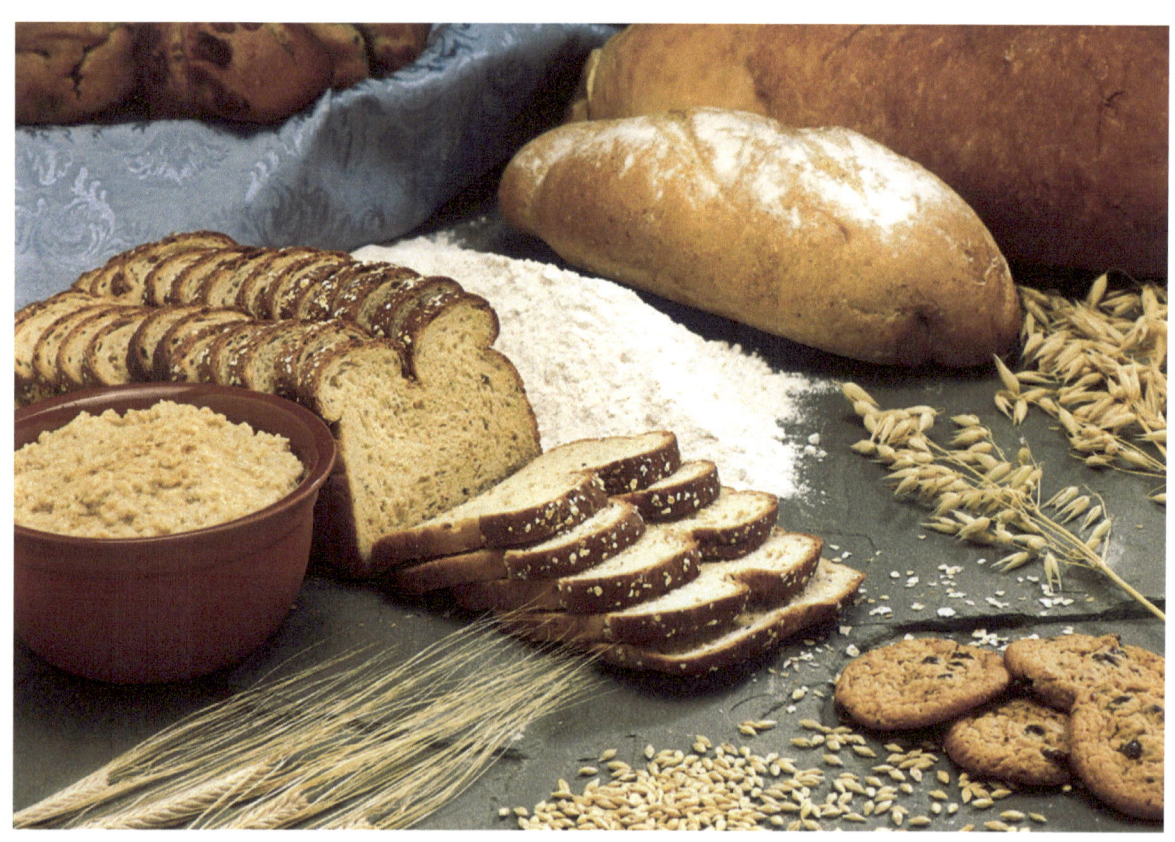

Whole oat grains have many wonderful benefits, which you can obtain by eating any food product that contains oats, as is the case with healthy and delicious oat bread.

Let us learn in the following the most important information about oat bread and the health benefits of oats:

What is oat bread?

Oat bread is made primarily from oat flour and a group of other various ingredients, such as: water, salt, and yeast .

Its benefits come from the high nutritional value of whole oat grains that are used to make and prepare this type of bread, as oats are rich in the following substances and nutrients:

A group of minerals, such as: magnesium, iron, and zinc.

Some types of vitamins, such as: vitamin B1 .

Dietary fiber.

One slice of whole grain oatmeal bread contains 130 calories, a good amount of carbohydrates and protein, and very little fat.

Benefits of oatmeal bread

The health benefits of oatmeal bread come from the whole grains of oats that are used in its manufacture, whether the oats used in it are in the form of flour or coarse whole grains . Here is a list of the most important benefits of oats and its bread:

1. Improving heart and arterial health

Regularly including whole grain oats in your diet may help improve the overall health of your circulatory system .

Whether you want to eat this type of grain by using its flour to make healthy bread or you want to mix it with milk for a healthy breakfast rich in energy and various nutrients, eating oats may help with the following:

Reducing high blood pressure levels .

Lowering cholesterol levels.

Reducing the chances of developing some heart and arterial diseases, especially coronary artery disease.

2. Cancer prevention

Oats and food products that contain oats, such as oat bread, may help reduce the chances of developing cancer, especially colorectal cancer, as oat grains contain nutritional elements that may help prevent inflammation, which may have a role in the development of various cancers.

3. Regulating blood sugar levels

Oats and food products made from oats may be a good choice for people with diabetes , as oats may help lower high blood sugar levels and regulate blood sugar, especially in people with type 2 diabetes.

4. Reduce weight

Because oats contain a relatively high amount of dietary fiber and some other important nutrients, eating it regularly may help reduce excess weight, by enhancing the feeling of satiety and curbing appetite in addition to improving the body's metabolism, and eating oats regularly may help reduce the chances of Obesity . _

5. Other benefits

Whole grain oats and oat products may have many other nutritional benefits, such as:

Boosting energy levels in the body, which may be particularly beneficial for those who exercise.

Strengthening the body's immunity .

Improve sleep quality.

Accelerate digestion, and prevent some digestive problems, such as: constipation and diarrhea.

How to make oatmeal bread at home
You can easily make bread at home by following these steps:

1. Necessary components

Here are the ingredients:

Half a cup of oats.
Half a cup of whole wheat flour.
A cup of boiling water.
A tablespoon of honey .
A tablespoon of oil.
A teaspoon of salt .
Two teaspoons of yeast.
2 cups of whole-grain flour made of any kind you like.

2. Preparation method

You can prepare oatmeal bread with these simple steps:

1-Mix wheat flour with oatmeal in a deep bowl.

2-Add boiling water, oil, salt, honey, and stir well.

3-Mix the yeast with a little warm water and sugar in a small cup.

4-Leave the mixture aside for 10 minutes until bubbles begin to appear on the surface of the mixture.

5-Add the yeast and water mixture to the bowl containing the rest of the ingredients and stir the mixture well.

6-Start adding the remaining two cups of flour to the mixture slowly, stirring well until you have a cohesive dough.

7-Leave the dough aside, covered, for at least an hour until it rises and doubles in size.

8-Spread the loaf of bread in the special oven tray.

9-Place it in the oven after sprinkling its outer surface with some whole oats.

10-Wait an hour for the loaf to cool after taking it out of the oven, then cut it and enjoy it.

When is oat bread not a healthy option?

There are different types of oat bread available in the market, which may seem healthy at first glance, but you must be careful and pay attention to the ingredients and the proportions of ingredients used to make the bread before choosing the appropriate type, as some manufactured types may contain the following:

Other types of processed and unhealthy flour.

Very low percentage of oats and oat flour compared to other ingredients in bread.

High content of: preservatives, sugars, and oils.

Gluten: Sometimes the oat crop may be mixed during cultivation or processing with wheat crops and other grains that contain gluten, so it should be eaten with caution by people who suffer from gluten allergy.

A delicious and healthy recipe for oatmeal cookies

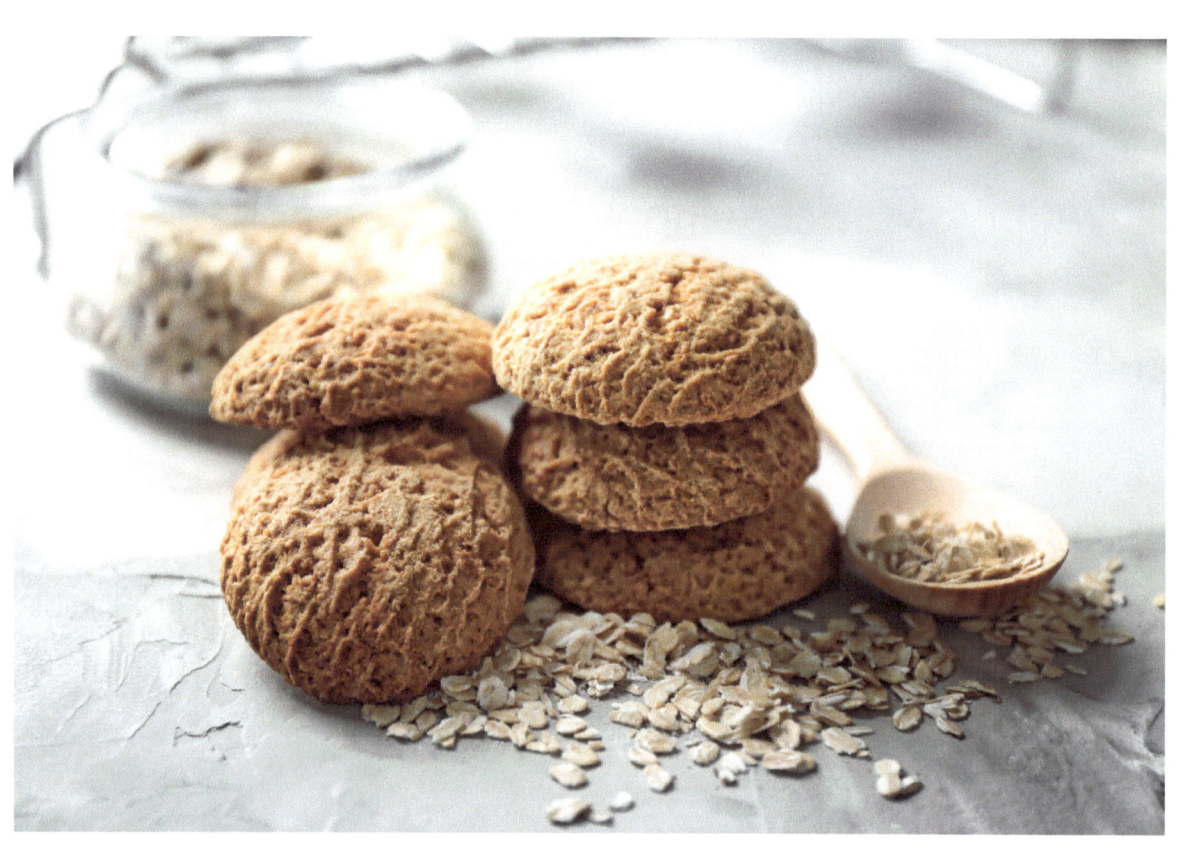

Here is a recipe for very useful oatmeal biscuits, especially as a breakfast meal for you and your children, and we are also pleased to remind you of the benefits of oatmeal for health.

In this article, we put in your hands a recipe for sugar-free oatmeal cookies, which is a healthy and very quick recipe to prepare, and we will also present the health benefits of oats, as desserts can be healthy and sometimes beneficial.

Recipe for healthy oatmeal cookies

Find out the details of a recipe for healthy oat biscuits below:

1. Ingredients and recipe for oat biscuits

To prepare a recipe for delicious oat biscuits, enough for approximately 24 biscuits, you will need:

2 cups of plain oats.

3 fruits of banana .

⅓ cup of natural apple juice.

½ cup of raisins (optional).

¼ cup of almond milk.

1 teaspoon of vanilla extract.

1 teaspoon of ground cinnamon .

2. Preparation method

Follow these easy steps to fully master the recipe, which takes 10 minutes to prepare and a quarter of an hour to bake, i.e. only 25 minutes :

1-Preheat the oven until it reaches 175°C.

2-Mash the bananas while the oven is preheating.

3-Mix all ingredients together in a bowl until you get a rough but homogeneous dough.

4-Scoop the mixture with a spoon and drop the ingredients onto the baking tray covered with baking paper without pressing the dough into the tray to flatten it.

5-Bake the tray ingredients until the edges of the product become golden, between 15-20 minutes.

3. Nutritional values in this recipe for oat biscuits

First, here is some nutritional value of the oat biscuits in this recipe as follows:

Nutritional valueQuantity: 1 biscuit	
energy52 calories	
Fats0.5 gr	
Carbohydrates11.2 grams	
Protein1.2 grams	
Sodium3 milligrams	
Cholesterol 0	

Tips for the success of the recipe for oatmeal cookies

Here are some tips that will help you make a successful oatmeal cookie recipe:

Make sure your recipe is reliable and that you follow the instructions carefully. If you miss an ingredient or any of the measurements, you could ruin the entire kit.

Check your baking equipment to be of high quality. Check your oven and adjust the preheat temperature 10–20 minutes before placing the baking tray.

Make sure the cookies are roughly evenly sized. You can buy an ice cream scoop to help get perfect portions of oatmeal cookie dough.

Make sure the ingredients are valid before using them and avoid using very old ingredients that have been stored for a long time in the kitchen.

What are the benefits of oats?

Here we remind you of some of the benefits that oats have for the health of you and your family members, and we are confident that you will be more excited to try a recipe for oat biscuits:

1. It benefits the heart and diabetes

Oats contain soluble fiber, which helps lower cholesterol levels and stabilize blood glucose levels. Therefore, oats protect the body from heart disease and diabetes.

2. Improves gut and digestive health

Oats also contain insoluble fiber, which is a slow-digesting fiber that promotes intestinal health and reduces constipation .

3. It protects against obesity

Whole oats and insoluble fiber occupy the stomach for a long time, which ensures a feeling of satiety for longer periods, helps control weight, and prevents obesity .

4. It is a storehouse of important minerals

Oatmeal provides a group of important minerals for the body, as it is rich in thiamine, magnesium, phosphorus, zinc, manganese, selenium, and iron.

5. A gluten-free feast

In its natural state, oatmeal is gluten-free, but you must be careful before buying it to ensure that no gluten-containing ingredients are added to it. The world of oatmeal manufacturing is very wide.

Oats and diabetes

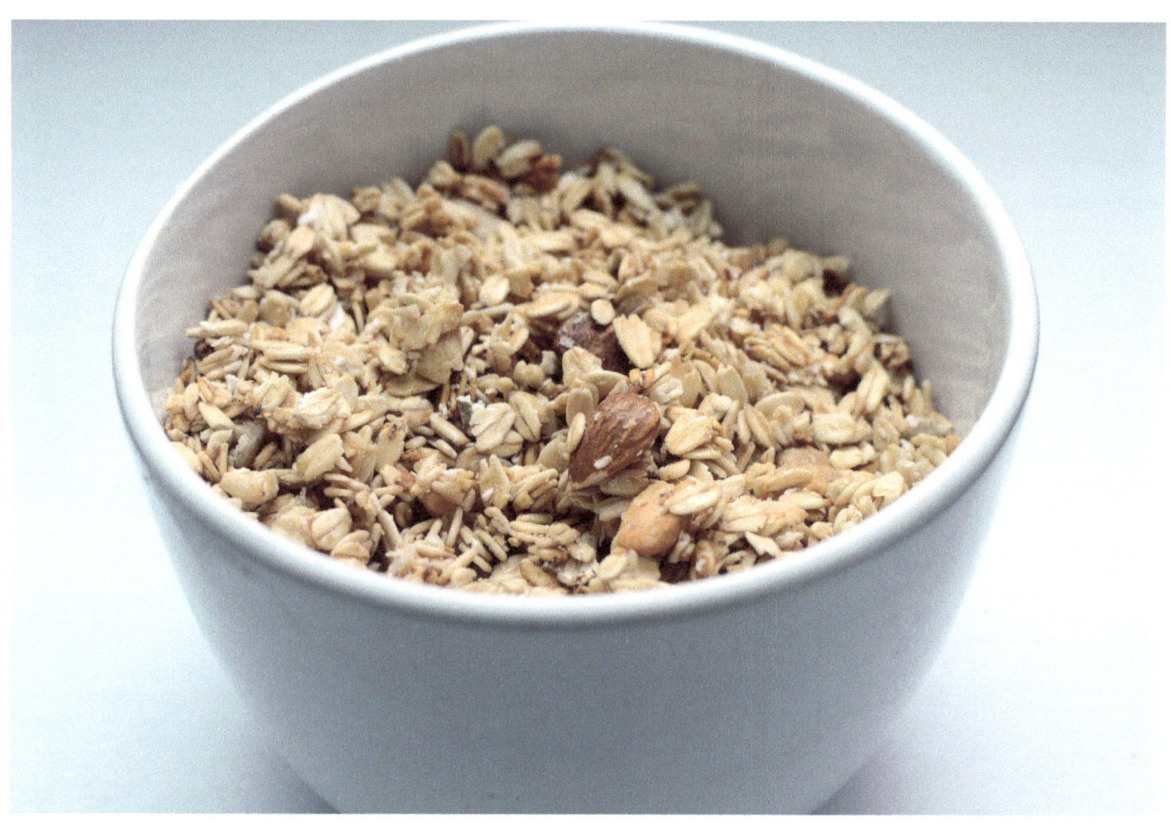

Oatmeal is a healthy breakfast option, but its carbohydrate content may worry diabetics, so what is the relationship between oatmeal and diabetes?

Long-term high blood sugar levels can cause long-term complications of diabetes to develop gradually.

The first step to controlling your blood sugar is to limit the amount of carbohydrates you eat because they directly affect blood sugar levels.

Here is an explanation of the relationship between oats and diabetes:

Oats and diabetes: the positives

It is preferable to choose types of carbohydrates that contain a low percentage of fats and sugars, which are matched by a high percentage of fiber and nutrients.

These specifications combine in oats to provide many health benefits for diabetics, with determining its quantities.

As oats offer many health benefits for diabetics, as long as their quantities are controlled, adding oats to the diet for diabetics provides the following advantages:

One of the most important advantages of oatmeal and diabetes is that one cup of cooked oats contains an amount of carbohydrates commensurate with the diabetic diet .

It can help regulate blood sugar levels, as it contains a moderate amount of fiber and a low glycemic index .

Oats are considered a heart-healthy food because they contain soluble fiber, such as beta-glucan, which has been linked to lower levels of bad cholesterol, blood sugar, and insulin.

It may reduce the need for multiple, high doses of insulin when eaten in place of breakfast foods that are high in carbohydrates and sugar.

It is a quick and easy meal to prepare.

It causes a feeling of satiety for a longer period and helps regulate weight, due to its high fiber content .

It contains a high percentage of soluble fiber, which increases the production of beneficial bacteria in the intestines that help in digestion.

It can be adopted as a fixed breakfast, because diabetics need to eat a fixed amount of carbohydrates every day, depending on diabetes medications or insulin type.

Oats and diabetes: the negatives

Oatmeal can lead to a higher blood sugar level than the normal limit for diabetics in the following cases:

Choose instant or quick oatmeal.

Choose the type of oatmeal that contains added sugar.

Eat a very large amount of oats.

Adding a large amount of dried fruits or sweeteners to the oatmeal.

Methods of preparing oats for diabetics

Oatmeal can be prepared with water, milk, or yogurt, or it can be eaten in the form of pancakes, cakes, or bread. Oatmeal can also be prepared and served to diabetics in different ways, some of which are mentioned below:

The first method: Mix one part of oatmeal with two parts of water or low-fat milk, and decorate the dish with some fruits and nuts.

Method 2: Mix oatmeal with water or yogurt and add vegetables or lean protein, such as grilled chicken, tomatoes or spinach, with a little lemon juice and olive oil

Information that may interest you about oats
Oatmeal is a type of cereal and is prepared by grinding the grains into a coarse powder.

The more processed the oats, such as processed oats and instant oats, the faster they are digested and the higher your blood sugar.

Therefore, whole grain oats are a better choice for diabetics because they contain vitamin B complex , proteins, calcium and fiber .

In addition, oats contain iron, manganese, potassium, magnesium, phosphorus, zinc, selenium and many other nutrients.

Benefits of oats
for the kidneys

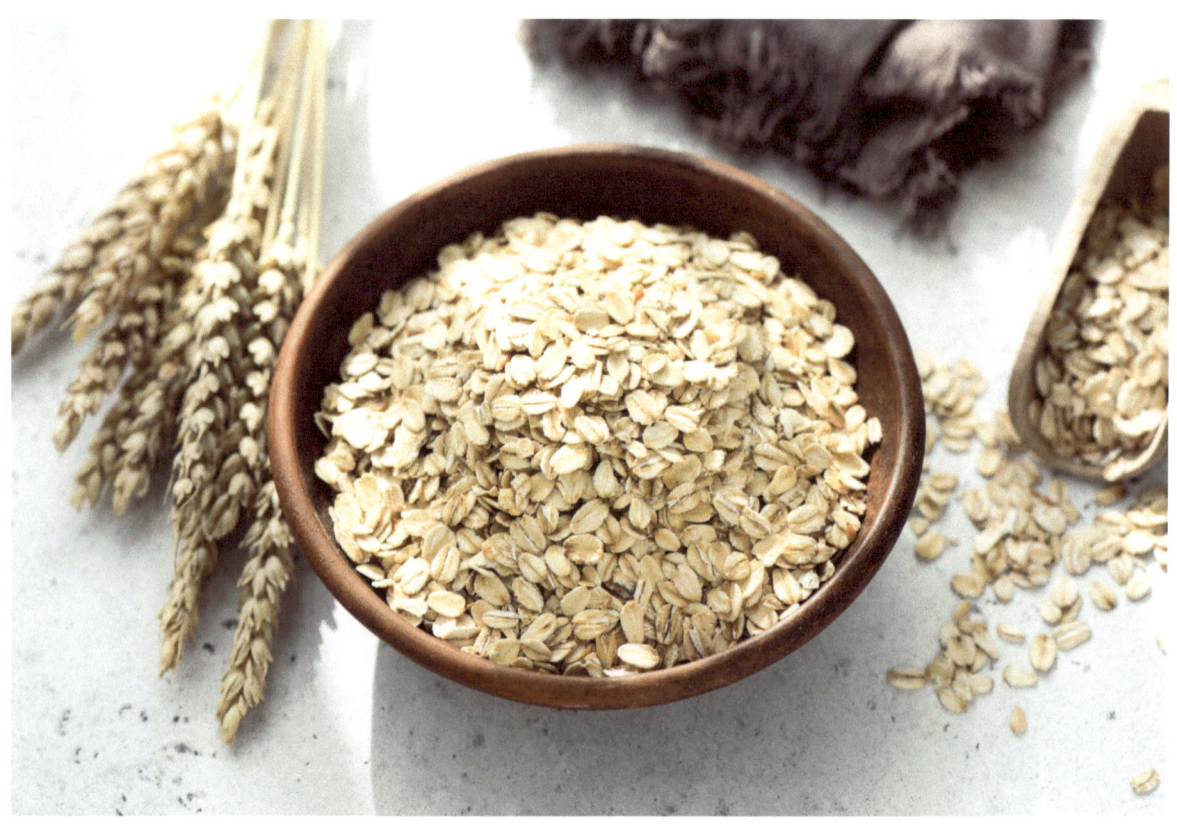

Oats contain many minerals and vitamins necessary for the body. Learn in this article about the benefits of oats specifically for the kidneys.

Below are the most prominent benefits of oats for the kidneys, the harms of excessive consumption, and important recommendations when eating oats for kidney patients:

Benefits of oats for the kidneys
Oats promote kidney health because they contain many vitamins and minerals, such as : vitamin B6, vitamin B3, copper, manganese, and iron.

One of its most prominent benefits for the kidneys is its positive effect on vital indicators of kidney function, which reduces the risk of kidney disease, as oats have a beneficial effect on the levels of albumin and potassium in the blood.

Other health benefits of oats

Among the other health benefits of oats that benefit all organs of the body, including the kidneys, and they also benefit specifically for kidney patients, we mention:

1. Promote a healthy body

Oats contain many important benefits and nutrients to enhance body health and increase energy, such as: iron, vitamin B1, pantothenic acid, and copper .

2. Improve digestive health

One of the most prominent benefits of oats for the kidneys is that it helps enhance the health of the digestive system, such as: improving the digestive process, regulating bowel movement, and promoting the growth of good bacteria in the intestine. It also helps reduce diseases and problems that may occur in the digestive tract and digestive system, such as: constipation. , and bloating.

3. Maintaining a healthy heart

Oats help maintain and promote heart health in kidney patients in particular, as oats contain soluble fiber, which sends signals to the liver to get rid of harmful cholesterol in the blood, which reduces the risk of atherosclerosis.

4. Reducing inflammation

Oats contain antioxidant properties, such as polyphenols, as they help reduce inflammation that may occur in the body.

5. Lowering blood sugar

Oatmeal lowers blood sugar levels by increasing insulin sensitivity, and this is one of the most important benefits of oats for kidney patients.

6. Lose weight

One of the most important benefits of oats is its role in losing weight, because it contains many nutrients, such as: zinc, magnesium, phosphorus, and fiber, as these elements help to feel full quickly and thus maintain a healthy weight and reduce excess weight.

The effects of overeating oats

After learning about the benefits of oats for the kidneys, here are some potential harms when eating too much oats:

Oats contain a high percentage of phosphorus , which may not be completely absorbed into the blood, so it may lead to increased pressure on kidney function, especially in people who suffer from chronic kidney disease.

Oats are very rich in fiber, and eating them frequently during the day may lead to a feeling of bloating.

Recommendations when eating oats
Here are some recommendations that are important
to know when eating oats:

It is recommended to avoid or limit the intake of
processed oats and replace them with natural oats:
such as whole oats or steel-cut oats, which take
longer to cook but are healthier because they contain
potassium, phosphorus, and sodium in a lower
percentage compared to processed oats. It is also
recommended to eat natural oats to avoid increasing
pressure on the functions. Kidneys, especially for
chronic kidney patients.
Some people suffer from an allergy when eating oats,
so you must ensure that there is no allergy before
eating it. Some people may also suffer from celiac
disease or an allergy to the gluten found in oats, so it
is recommended to eat oats that do not contain
gluten to prevent and avoid the effects. collateral.

Oatmeal is one of the types of cereals rich in nutrients and health benefits. But does it have any harm for men? Let's find out how much oatmeal is really harmful to men in this article.

Oats (Avena sativa) is a species of cereal in the family Poaceae (Poaceae). The oat plant consists of oat seeds, leaves and stems, i.e. oat straw, and bran, which is the outer layer of the entire oat. These different parts of the plant are used to make medicinal herbal supplements.

Oats are one of the most nutritious foods served at breakfast, as they help maintain vitality and activity, increase attention span, and improve mental performance.

Some people wonder what the harmful effects of oatmeal are for men specifically. Are there any actual harms? Here's the answer:

Oatmeal damage to mendoes it really exist?

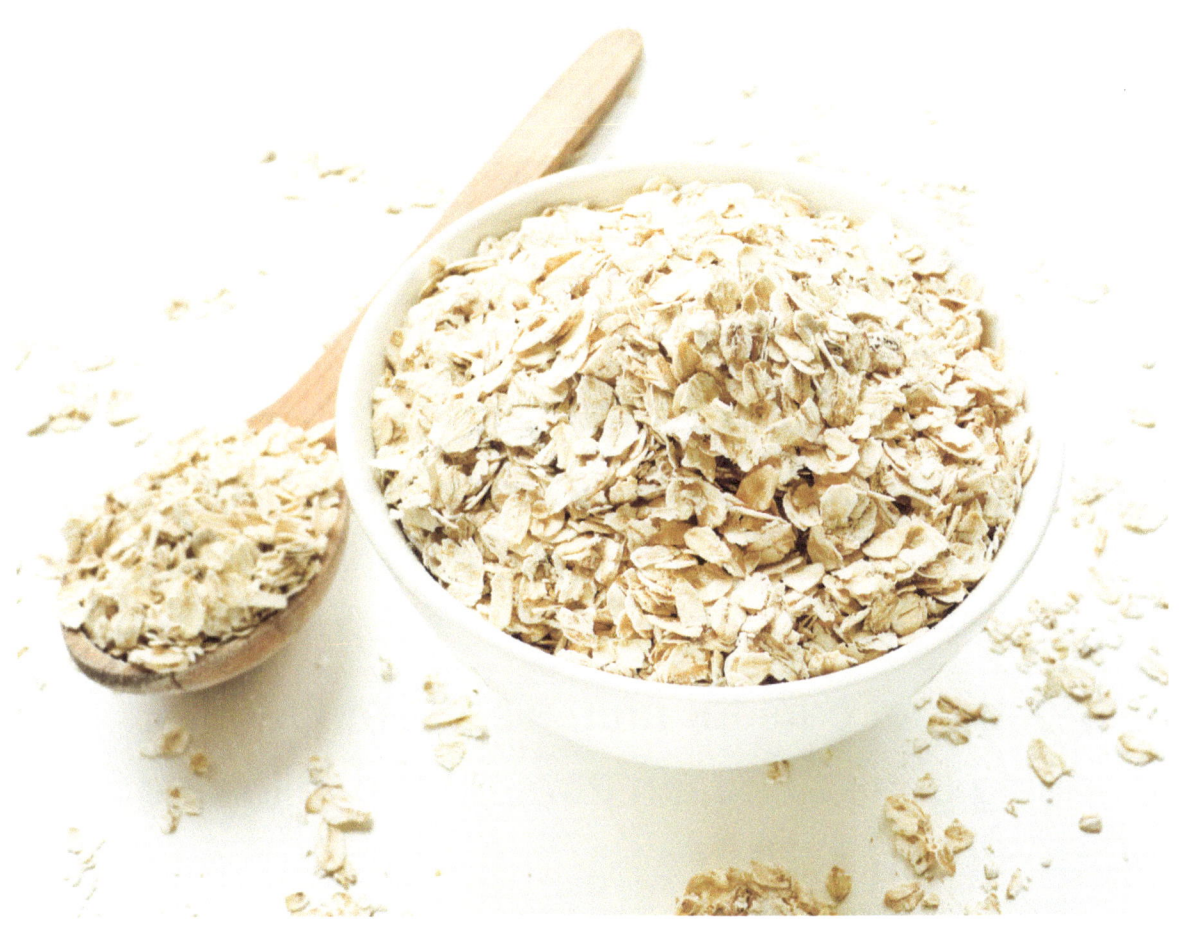

Oatmeal damage to men: is it real?

In fact, there is no harm to men from oats, as oats may contribute to enhancing their sexual health through the following:

Oats help men reach orgasm as they are a source of aphrodisiac.

Oats contain the amino acid L-arginine, which helps the blood vessels in the penis to relax, which is necessary for a man to maintain an erection and reach orgasm.

Improves testosterone level and increase libido.

It helps in sperm formation, thanks to the zinc found in oats, which plays an important role in this.

Studies have not proven that oats are harmful to men in particular with regard to sexual health.

The benefits of oats for men also contribute to enhancing general health through the following:

The antioxidants in oats play an effective role in preventing heart disease.

The dietary fiber contained in oats helps lower levels of bad cholesterol (LDL) without affecting levels of good cholesterol (HDL).

Oats help enhance the immune response to diseases because they contain beta-glucan.

It helps protect the skin, as oatmeal has been used as a soothing agent to relieve itching and irritation. In addition, it helps moisturize and soften the skin.

Beta-glucan fiber found in oats helps control blood sugar and insulin levels after a meal.

It helps in weight control as beta-glucan fibers attract water, which increases the viscosity of digested food and the volume of food in the digestive tract.

It slows digestion and the rate of absorption of nutrients, which in turn increases the sense of satiety.

Helps maintain a healthy digestive system as fiber contributes to bowel regularity and prevention of constipation. It also has the ability to increase the weight and water content of stool, making it easier to pass.

General oat damage

After identifying the harms of oats for men, we note that the harms of oats in general include the following:

Flatulence .

anal irritation

Skin irritation when using topical products containing oatmeal.

Contraindications for the use of oats

To avoid exposure to the harms of oats for men and women, you must refrain from using oats according to the following:

People with celiac disease or other disorders of the digestive system.

People with intestinal obstruction, including: the esophagus, stomach, and intestines.

People who suffer from slow digestion.

Children with atopic dermatitis may have an increased risk of oat allergy.

Learn about the benefits of oats for women

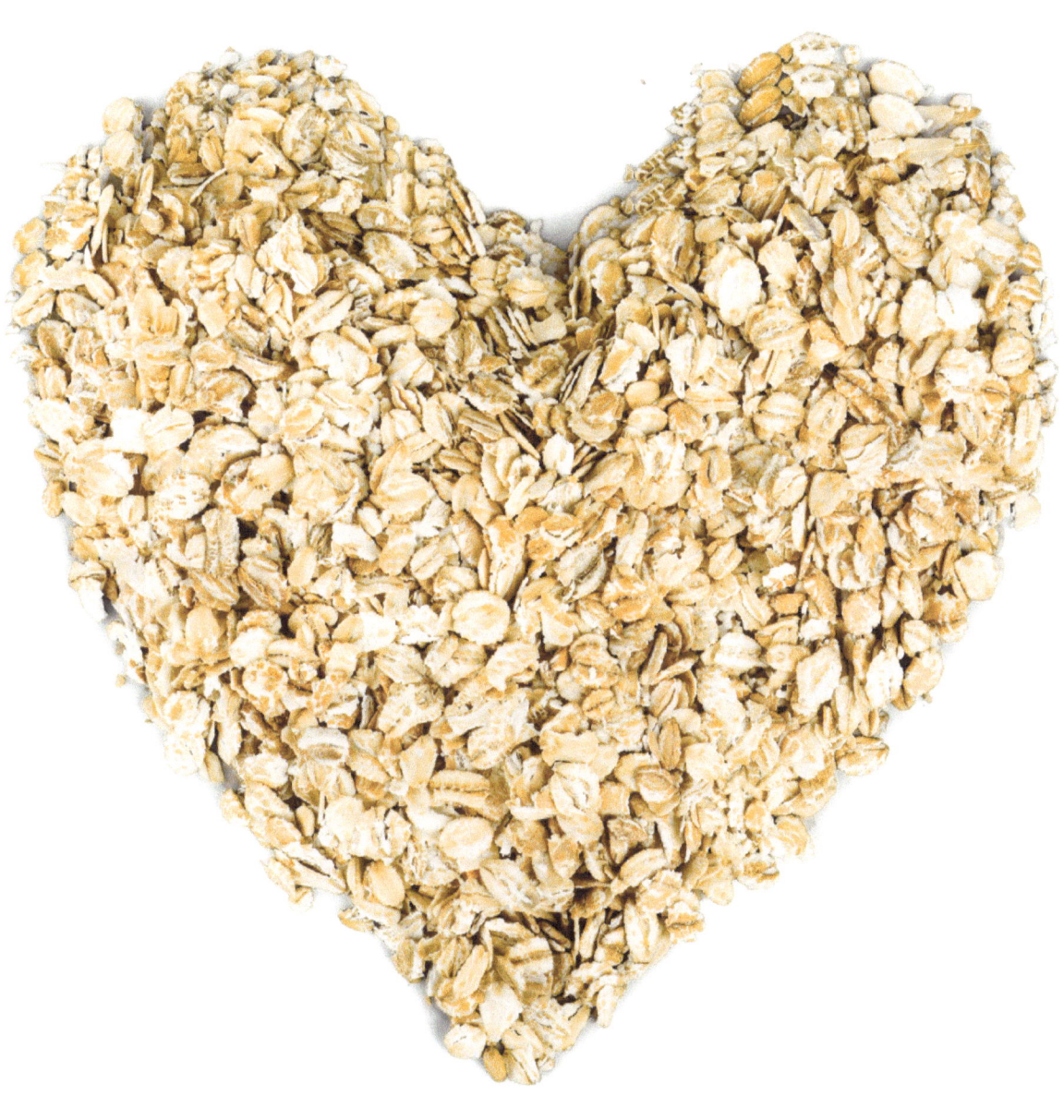

Oatmeal has many benefits for women and others, so what are the benefits of oatmeal for women specifically?

Oats is one of the whole grains with many health benefits, because it contains a number of essential elements and antioxidants that may benefit women in particular, which makes it one of the meals that is recommended to be added to the diet. Continue reading the following article to learn more about the benefits of oats for women:

Benefits of oats for women
Oatmeal is characterized by its delicious taste and ease of cooking with different meals or even with desserts, in addition to its proposed health benefits that may be of particular interest to women. Here are the most prominent benefits of oatmeal for women:

1. Helping you lose weight

Oatmeal is an excellent addition to any diet aimed at losing or maintaining weight, due to its richness in dietary fibers such as beta-glucan, which works to absorb the water present in the meal eaten, thus increasing the volume of the meal in the stomach, which leads to an increase in Sense of fullness and reduce the feeling of hunger.

2. Maintaining a healthy digestive system

Dietary fibers, both soluble and insoluble in water, maintain normal bowel movement and reduce constipation, which is a problem that many women suffer from, especially during pregnancy.

In addition, these fibers, including beta-glucan, ferment in the intestine and thus maintain the health of the beneficial bacteria in it, which have a major role in maintaining the health of the digestive system and relieving the symptoms of Irritable Bowel Syndrome, such as: diarrhea, constipation, and bloating ..

Many vitamins and antioxidants in oats also prevent cancer, especially colon cancer.

3. Reducing the symptoms of Celiac disease

Celiac disease is one of the immune diseases that occurs at a higher rate in women, as the incidence of it in women may be three times higher than that in men.

People with celiac disease need to follow a special gluten-free diet, so oatmeal is one of the excellent alternatives to being gluten-free, and it can also be used in the form of flour to prepare bread, cakes, or pastries of all kinds.

It is worth noting that although oats are gluten-free, they may cause sensitivity in some people with celiac disease, so it is important to consult a doctor before adding them to the diet.

4. Prevention of chronic diseases

Oatmeal is one of the food sources that have a suggested role in preventing many chronic diseases that some women may suffer from as they age, as oats reduce harmful cholesterol in the body and prevent high pressure.

Oats also reduce the sudden rise in blood sugar after eating, and improve tissue sensitivity to insulin, which may have benefits for people with type 2 diabetes .

5. Reducing skin inflammation

Some studies indicate the role of oatmeal and the skin care products that contain it in reducing the symptoms of dermatitis, such as: redness and itching associated with a number of skin diseases, such as: eczema, dryness, and skin irritation.

This is due to its richness in antioxidants that are beneficial to the skin, such as vitamin E and the anti-inflammatory compound avenanthramides.

Benefits of oats for pregnant women
Oatmeal is one of the safe and excellent foods for use by pregnant women. Here are the most important benefits of oatmeal for pregnant women:

It is a food source rich in complex carbohydrates, which provides pregnant women with energy and activity during the day.

It contains a number of vitamins and essential elements during pregnancy for the health of the mother and fetus, most notably iron, zinc, magnesium, manganese, potassium, calcium, in addition to folic acid.

It plays a role in preventing the occurrence of gestational diabetes because it contains fiber and complex carbohydrates that work to prevent a sudden rise in blood sugar after meals.

It prevents common constipation in pregnant women as it contains dietary fiber.

It is an excellent meal for pregnant women during the first months of pregnancy, when women may suffer from nausea and difficulty eating certain foods.

Oats side effects

After we got acquainted with the most important benefits of oats for women, here are the most prominent possible side effects that may occur as a result of eating oats:

The possibility of bloating because oats contain fiber, especially if you eat large amounts of it, but this symptom often disappears with time.

Causing indigestion and diarrhea when taken in large quantities.

Some people experience hypersensitivity symptoms if they are allergic to oats.

Oatmeal for the facebenefits and recipes

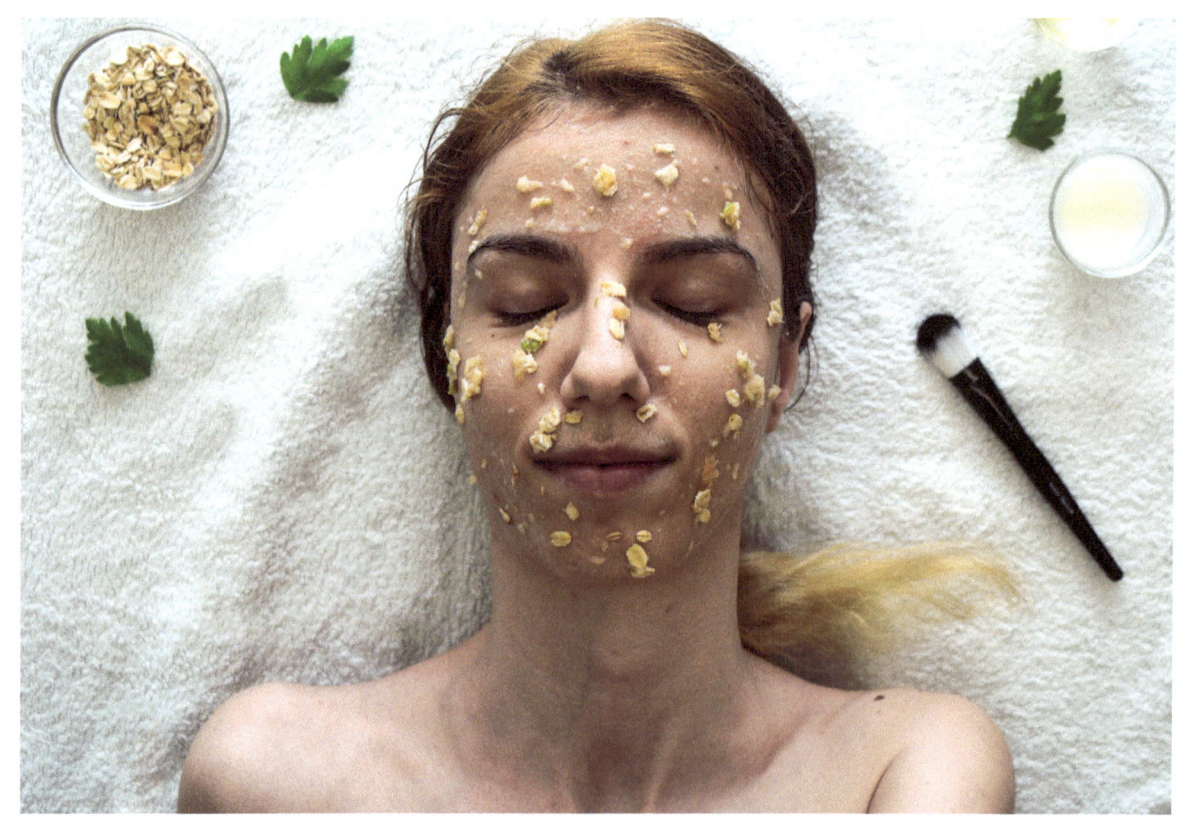

It is hardly hidden from one of the many and many benefits of oatmeal in general for health, so what are the benefits of oatmeal for the face specifically? Here are the most important ones in this article.

Oats have many and varied health benefits in general, and wonderful benefits for the skin and for the face in particular. Here are the most important benefits of oats for the face in the following article:

Benefits of oatmeal for the face

Learn about a group of oatmeal benefits for the face and recipes to obtain these benefits through the following:

Acne Treatment

Oatmeal helps absorb excess fat in the skin and treat and control acne . To benefit from oatmeal for the face in this case, follow these steps:

Boil a third of a cup of water with half a cup of oats for a little while.
Leave the mixture to cool slightly.
Apply the mixture on the face, and make it thicker, especially in the areas affected by acne.
Leave the mixture on the face for 20 minutes, then wash it off with warm water.

Removal of dead cells

You can also benefit from oatmeal for the face as well, by making a quick and effective scrub to get rid of dead skin cells. This is how it works:

Benefits of oatmeal for the face

Learn about a group of oatmeal benefits for the face and recipes to obtain these benefits through the following:

Acne Treatment

Oatmeal helps absorb excess fat in the skin and treat and control acne . To benefit from oatmeal for the face in this case, follow these steps:

1-Boil a third of a cup of water with half a cup of oats for a little while.

2-Leave the mixture to cool slightly.

3-Apply the mixture on the face, and make it thicker, especially in the areas affected by acne.

4-Leave the mixture on the face for 20 minutes, then wash it off with warm water.

Removal of dead cells

You can also benefit from oatmeal for the face as well, by making a quick and effective scrub to get rid of dead skin cells. This is how it works:

1-Mix a teaspoon of ground oatmeal with a teaspoon of natural honey, a teaspoon of jojoba oil, and a few drops of lavender oil .

2-Apply the mixture to wet facial skin, distribute it well, and then gently rub the skin with circular motions.

3-Leave the mixture on the face for 10 minutes.

4-Wash off the mixture with warm water and then gently dry your face.

It is worth noting that several types of face washes and scrubs rich in oatmeal are available in the market.

Moisturizing the skin

Regular use of oatmeal for the face, in particular, helps to get rid of dead cells and prevent their accumulation, thus helping the skin to maintain its moisture naturally.

To get the benefits of oatmeal for the face in this case, follow these steps:

1-Mix two cups of oats with one cup of milk and one tablespoon of honey.
2-Apply the resulting mixture to the skin of the face.
3-Leave the mixture on the face for 15 minutes.
4-Wash your face with warm water.
Delaying signs of aging
Due to the exfoliating and antioxidant properties of oatmeal , using oatmeal for the face regularly helps to reverse the harmful effects of sunlight and delay the signs of skin aging.

Skin whitening
Because of the many benefits that oatmeal brings to the face in particular and to the skin in general, you can also use oatmeal to lighten facial skin.

For the purpose of lightening the skin , you just have to mix the oatmeal powder with milk and use it to wash the face every morning.

Sunburn treatment

It is possible to use oats to treat sunburn effectively, due to the moisturizing, antioxidant and soothing properties of oats.

Cleansing the skin naturally

One of the benefits of oatmeal for the face is that it can be used as a natural skin cleanser that removes impurities, dirt and oils from the skin.

To take advantage of oats for this purpose, here are the following methods:

1-Prepare oat milk by soaking oatmeal in water for a while, and then wipe the face with the resulting milk after washing your face.

2-Extracting oat milk by placing the oats inside a filtered piece of cloth, and exposing this piece to hot steam with a little pressure to get the resulting milk out of the pores of the cloth.

Other benefits of oatmeal for the face

Oatmeal has many other benefits for the face, here are the most important of them:

1-Helping sensitive skin , oatmeal is generally suitable for all skin types, and especially helps to relieve any irritation or sensitivity.

2-Clearing the skin, removing dead skin cells, and getting rid of blackheads.

3-A natural remedy for eczema , as it helps in some cases to control it.

4-Getting rid of acne scars and treating them.

5-Relieve itchy skin.

Side effects of using oatmeal on the face

Although oatmeal is considered safe and beneficial for the face, there are cases in which it was found that oatmeal contributed to irritating acne, so you should consult a doctor first before using it to treat your acne conditions.

People who are allergic to oatmeal should not use it on the face, and if you experience unwanted symptoms after using oatmeal on the face, such as: burning, rash, or stinging, stop using it and see your doctor immediately.

Benefits of oats for hair

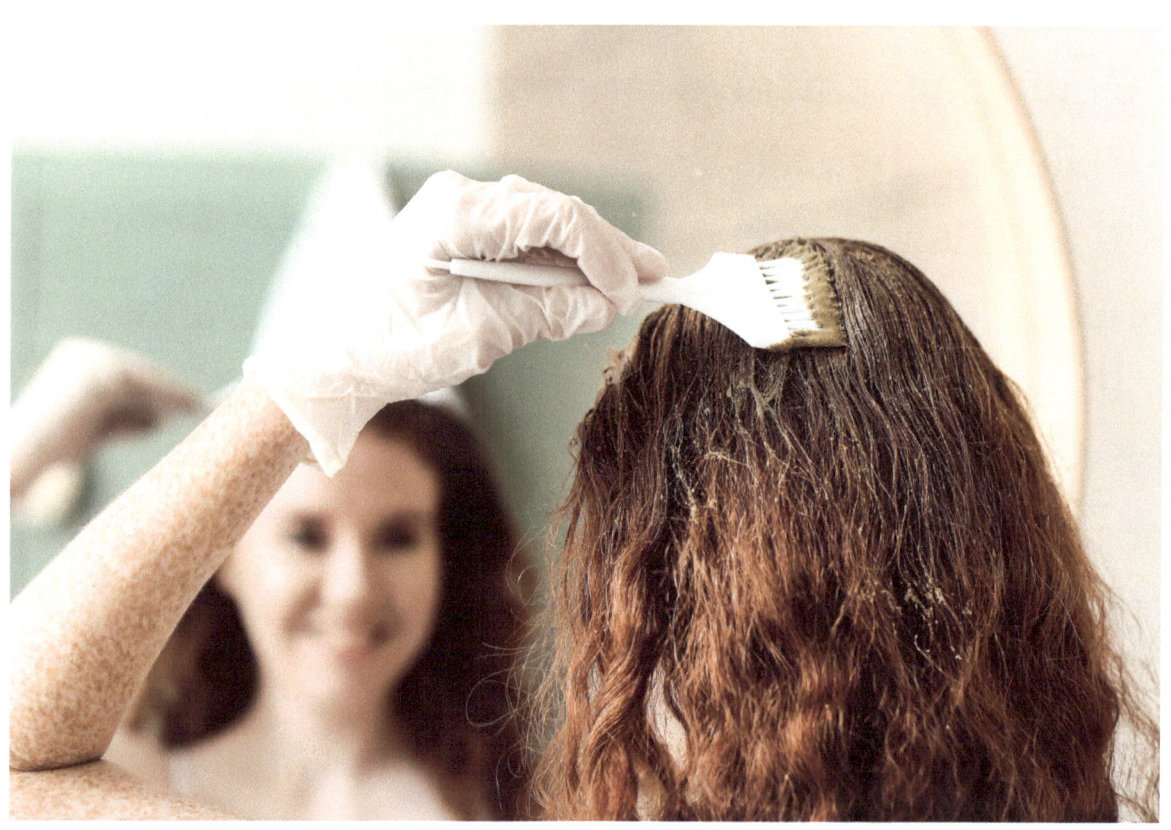

What are the benefits of oatmeal for hair? What are the ways in which oatmeal masks can be prepared? Here are the details in this article.

Oatmeal is included in the preparation of both skin and hair products due to the valuable benefits it provides, and in this article we will discuss the benefits of oatmeal for hair in particular:

Benefits of oats for hair

The most important benefits of oats for hair include the following:

1. Prevents hair loss and improves hair growth

Oatmeal can help prevent hair loss thanks to its high fiber content that promotes scalp health, in addition to its gentle exfoliating properties that open the scalp pores and facilitate hair growth.

2. Prevents split ends of hair

Damage to the ends of the hair spoils the overall appearance of the hair, and therefore it must be treated immediately to keep the hair vibrant and healthy. Oatmeal provides an excellent option for treating the problem of split ends, as it is rich in vitamins and minerals that give the hair the moisture and nutrition it needs to remain healthy from the roots to the ends .

3. Treats dandruff

Oats contain a high percentage of proteins and fats that give the scalp the moisture it needs to avoid the appearance of dandruff

4. Soothes dry scalp

The problem of dry scalp is accompanied by itching and irritation, which causes discomfort and anxiety. To get rid of these problems, oats can be used as they contain a high percentage of vitamin B, which gives the scalp the moisture it needs and locks in moisture.

In addition, oats have anti-inflammatory properties that reduce scalp itching and prevent irritation.

5. Improves the appearance of hair

Oatmeal adds shine and softness to the hair strands, making the hair as a whole look healthy and elegant.

6. It is used to care for blonde hair

People with blonde hair may find it difficult to find hair products that help care for their hair and maintain its beauty without harming the health of the hair, while oatmeal provides all of this without causing any significant damage.

Ways to use oatmeal for hair

After we learned about the benefits of oatmeal for hair, we must learn about ways to benefit from it:

1. Oatmeal and apple cider vinegar mask

This mask is used to treat the problem of itchy scalp and dandruff. It can be prepared by mixing 1 cup of oats until it becomes smooth, then adding 2 cups of boiling water and stirring the ingredients well, then leaving it aside for 10 minutes and then filtering it.

Add 1 teaspoon of apple cider vinegar, 1 tablespoon of lemon juice, and 20 drops of essential oil, then wet the hair with warm water and massage the mixture into the scalp, and rinse well after two minutes.

2. Oatmeal and coconut oil mask

This mask is prepared by adding 1/2 cup of milk to 3 tablespoons of oats, and stir together to obtain a paste, then add 1 tablespoon of coconut oil and 1 tablespoon of honey and stir well, then apply it to the hair and leave it for 30 minutes. Then rinse it with warm water.

3. Oatmeal and aloe vera gel mask
Grind 1/2 cup of oats to obtain a fine powder, then add 1 cup of milk, 1 teaspoon of olive oil, and 1 tablespoon of aloe vera gel, then rub the mask on the scalp for 5 minutes and leave it for at least an hour before rinsing the hair . .

Oatmeal damage to hair
In addition to applying it topically, oats can also be eaten to obtain its benefits for the hair. In both cases, it causes some side effects, the most notable of which are:

Digestive disorders and digestive problems.
Oat allergy, especially in people with atopic dermatitis.
Anal irritation .
Bloating and gas.

Oat allergy most important information

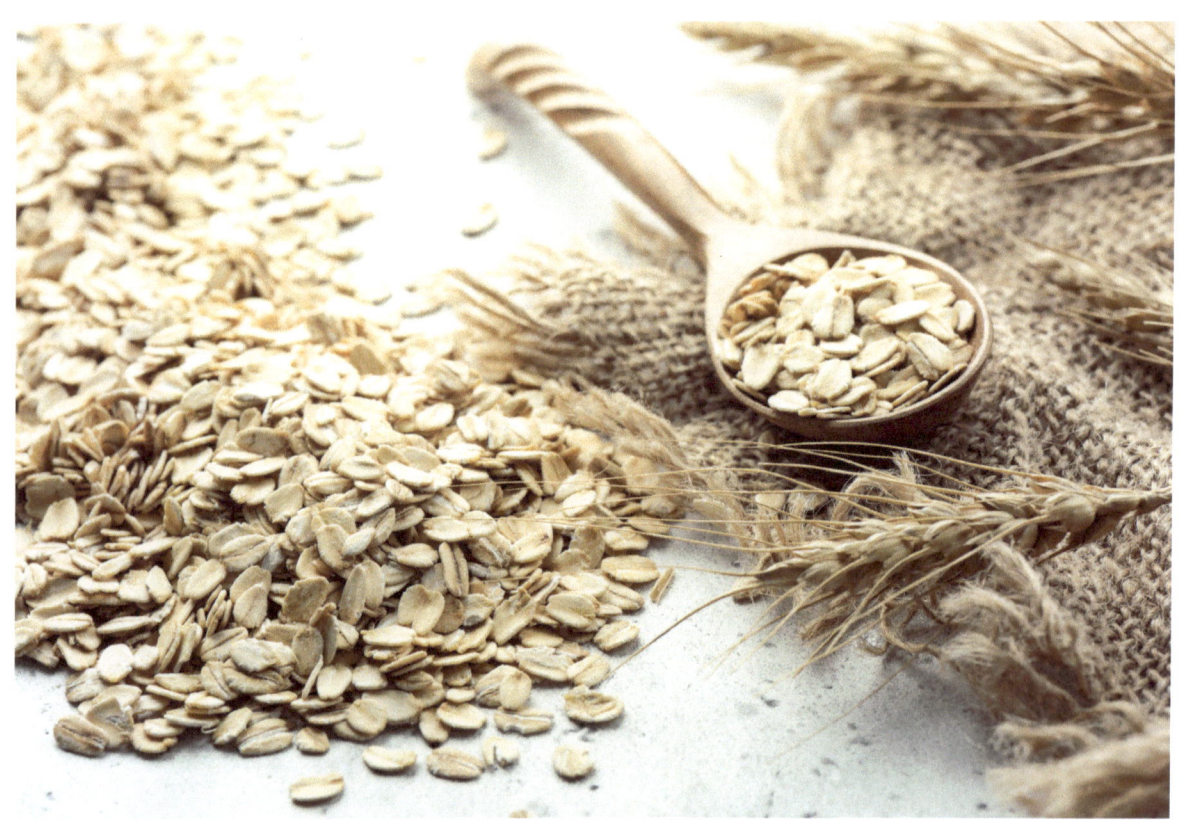

Have you felt unwell after eating a meal containing oats? You may have an oat allergy. What is this allergy? Find out the answer in this article.

Oats are usually grown and processed alongside wheat and other grains that contain gluten , which is an allergen for some, so the body's allergic reaction to oats may be due to cross-contamination with gluten, but in other cases the individual is allergic to the oats themselves. What is an oat allergy? Follow the following article with us:

Oat allergy and its symptoms

Oat allergy is the immune system's response to one of the oat proteins known as avenin. The body produces antibodies to fight this protein, thinking that it is a harmful substance to the body, which causes an allergic reaction when eating oats in individuals who are allergic to it. This allergy appears on the skin. Form a group of the following symptoms:

1. Mild symptoms of oat allergy

Like any other type of food allergy, the degree, severity, and nature of the allergy vary. Symptoms of the allergy may be mild and usually appear immediately after eating oats or within approximately two hours, and include the following:

Feeling itchy and tingling in the throat.
Watery and itchy eyes, runny nose and sneezing.
Redness and congestion of the face, swelling and sometimes puffiness of the lips and eyes.

A skin rash and itching appears around the mouth, tongue, and sometimes the eyes, and it may spread to other areas of the body.

An allergic reaction and itchy rash on the skin occurs after using topical products containing oats.

2. Symptoms of moderate severity of oat allergy

These symptoms also occur directly, but their severity is higher than the previous ones. Symptoms of moderate oat allergy include the following:

Exhaustion .

Bloating and stomach pain.

Nausea, vomiting and diarrhea.

3. Serious symptoms of oat allergy

Oat allergy can lead to symptoms of hypersensitivity (Anaphylaxis), which is a serious condition that requires an immediate visit to a doctor, as it can pose a threat to a person's life. These symptoms appear within an hour of exposure to oats and include the following:

Acceleration or weakness of the heartbeat.

Tightness in the chest and difficulty breathing .

Sudden drop in blood pressure.

Hearing sounds and whistling when breathing.

dizziness , confusion, or loss of consciousness;

4. Late symptoms of oat allergy

Some symptoms of oat allergy can appear late, that is, after 4-6 hours or more, and permanent exposure to oats may cause chronic diseases, and these symptoms include the following:

exhaustion.

diarrhea.

Inflammation and irritation of the stomach .

Food protein-induced enterocolitis syndrome-FPIES, symptoms include vomiting, dehydration, diarrhea, and growth problems.

How is oat allergy diagnosed?

Oat allergy can be diagnosed by a blood test, but it is inaccurate and the doctor resorts to it in the event that one of the other methods of diagnosis is not possible, and among these methods are the following:

1. Food challenge test

In this test, the doctor gives you small amounts of oats, gradually increasing them, and monitoring the body's reaction to them. The doctor can also determine whether your oat allergy is due to it containing gluten due to cross-contamination, or whether you have an allergy to the oat protein itself.

2. Skin prick test

The doctor uses a scalpel to expose the skin to a group of different allergens in small quantities and monitors the body's reaction to each of them in the area. This painless test takes approximately 20–40 minutes and is performed on the forearm area.

3. Patch test

This test is used to diagnose a delayed oat allergy. A patch containing the oat allergen is stuck to either the hand or back for about two days, after which the doctor checks the body's reaction to these patches.

Treatment of oat allergy

Like any other type of food allergy, the treatment is to avoid eating it, in addition to other methods that can be resorted to in the event of exposure to allergy symptoms. We explain the treatment of oat allergy as follows:

1. Avoid foods that contain oats

To avoid developing symptoms of oat allergy, you should read the ingredients of foods and avoid any type that contains oats. You should also avoid the following foods:

Oats, oatcakes and oat milk.
Granola and porridge.
Bathing products and creams containing oatmeal.

2. Treatment with medications

If an allergic reaction occurs in the body, your doctor may prescribe one of the following medications for you:

Antihistamine medications to relieve mild allergy symptoms.

Corticosteroid sprays to treat breathing-related symptoms.

Epinephrine self-injections are used in emergency situations when serious hypersensitivity symptoms occur.

**Prepare and compose
Professor / Radwan Abu Bakr
All copyrights reserved to the
author .© 2023**

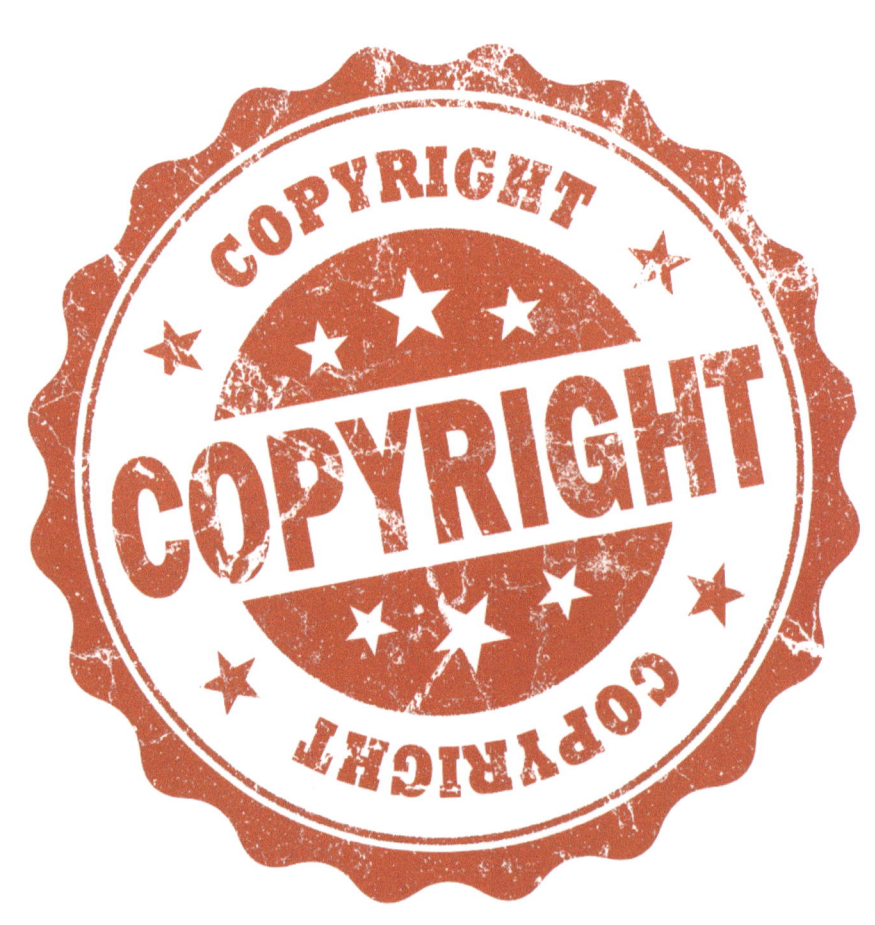

www.ingramcontent.com/pod-product-compliance
Lightning Source LLC
Chambersburg PA
CBHW041457280526
45792CB00004B/1043